# UNLOCKING WOMEN'S HEALTH

## FemTech and the Quest for Gender Equity

Foreword by Ida Tin,
co-founder of Clue

DR. BRITTANY BARRETO

*Unlocking Women's Health: FemTech and the Quest for Gender Equity*



In this world of digital information and rapidly-changing technology, some citations do not provide exact page numbers or credit the original source. We regret any errors, which are a result of the ease with which we consume information.

This content is based on interviews with experts on the *FemTech Focus* podcast. There are no citations for the statistics originally provided by the interviewees and any information should be confirmed by the reader.

The information provided in this book is strictly for informational purposes and is not intended as a substitute for advice from your physician or mental health provider. You should not use this information for diagnosis or treatment of any physical or mental health problem.

Editor: Laurie Knight
Developmental Editor: Amy Delcambre
Cover Design: Kristina Edstrom

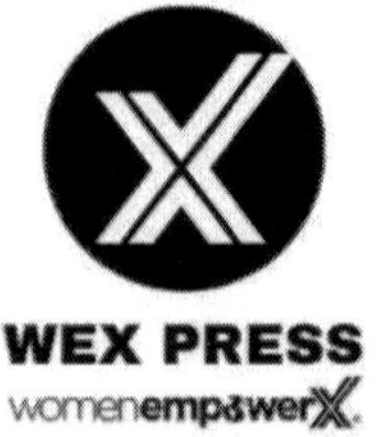


An Imprint for GracePoint Publishing (www.GracePointPublishing.com)
GracePoint Matrix, LLC
624 S. Cascade Ave, Suite 201, Colorado Springs, CO 80903
www.GracePointMatrix.com Email: Admin@GracePointMatrix.com
SAN # 991-6032

A Library of Congress Control Number has been requested and is pending.
ISBN: (Paperback) 978-1-961347-91-5
eISBN: 978-1-961347-92-2

Books may be purchased for educational, business, or sales promotional use.
For bulk order requests and price schedule contact: Orders@GracePointPublishing.com

This book is dedicated to every woman, female, and girl past and present who was in pain, sick, or died from unnecessary or preventable conditions.

Your pain is real.

You are not the only one.

You deserve to feel well.

May this book be a cornerstone of the movement that prevents future generations from this needless suffering.

# Table of Contents

# Foreword

**IT WAS NOT A GIVEN** that I'd found a technology company. I thought I'd be an artist. But then I realized something was missing in the world. Something I urgently needed. And I understood that literally billions of others were lacking it too—a type of birth control that didn't make you either hurt or sick or depressed, or all three. I decided to build one myself, prompted by smartphones and data as the tools at hand.

This was in 2008. Fast forward to 2016 and I'm deep in. As CEO and cofounder of a startup building an app called Clue—a period tracking app, a first step on my ambitious plan towards a new type of family planning method. Together with four men I founded the company in Berlin, and we have raised millions in venture funding. And as we do all this, I see other founders, mostly women, innovating in women's health too. That is fantastic news. I want us all to be understood as one, big, unstoppable movement in culture and in technology—all building FemTech! I know we need a word that can unite us, and most importantly help the world understand that we are not each—individually—building niche products, but collectively taking on the huge, overlooked, under researched, and underfunded task of moving female health into the digital age, to have women's bodies be cared for in a healthcare system that forgot us, ignored us, or actually did nasty things *to* us because of outdated cultural and gender ideas.

It's now a fact that FemTech is a force, fueled by real needs, by creativity and also by anger. Women are tired of waiting for the solutions they need. Now we build them ourselves. And, yes we are building! Despite funding still being unfairly hard to get, of all the usual struggles of being a working mum, of platforms censoring our ads as "adult content" and countless other obstacles, FemTech is on the rise. This is true around the planet from Africa to Japan, India, the Americas, and Europe. More venture capital is earmarked for female health than ever before, as is public funding. Accelerators, newsletters, and agencies are specializing in FemTech.

Brittany is one of these bright energy explosions moving this industry forward. With her background as a medical professional, she looks clear-eyed into this landscape of female healthcare. She is paving the way for people to understand what FemTech is and the potential it holds. The podcast and platform she built helps orient the ones innovating in this space. She has proven herself a valued resource for the wider community and a sharp and courageous voice reaching into the political system, to the corporate world, and to the medical world to rally us all toward better outcomes for female health.

And most importantly, women—whether we call ourselves users, customers, or patients—are starting to *expect* better care. It takes seven years to get diagnosed with endometriosis—a condition that isn't exactly rare (one out of twelve women suffer from it)—and that is unacceptable. Neither is stigmatizing menopause. Something that every single woman on the planet either has gone through, is in, or will go through cannot be a taboo, that is just absurd—and yet it is our reality. Now, luckily as the cultural notions shift and expand, so do the technological innovations. What culturally becomes possible paves the way for technical innovation. That is why it is so important for women to use their voices and to tell of their lived experiences. That is how we move forward.

I am so excited for this book doing just that—giving voice to FemTech. I believe we need to build bridges between the genders: We need men to understand what it means to have a female body. And with FemTech, we not only educate ourselves, but we also gather data that men can understand, do research on, fund, and innovate from. We need all genders to participate in FemTech; there is still much work to be done. And that also means there are great business opportunities waiting to be unfolded. We need the founders, but we also need the funders. And we need many more people—the fantastic teams, the lawyers, the journalists, the branding agencies. As we build our services and companies, let's build with diverse teams. This book is helping us achieve just that. I think of it as an invitation for the world to participate in FemTech. If you are not sure how, this book is for you. The book is a wonderful amplification of all of Brittany's work, and allows everyone to know what she learned over many years.

The book is a tour de force through all major areas of FemTech and some of the innovators building in the many areas of this large industry, where so many needs, ideas, and solutions are coming forth. I learned a lot reading this book, and I am sure many will be inspired by seeing this vast landscape of FemTech laid out with such clarity. It is an important book, showing both the painful gaps of female health and the huge potential there is in FemTech.

*Ida Tin, Co-founder of Clue*
*Coined the term FemTech in 2016*

# Introduction

**SHE WAS WELL PAST NINE MONTHS PREGNANT**, and her husband demanded the physician deliver the baby. The doctor finally obliged and took the patient in for a cesarean. But when they cut her open, they found a dead, stillborn baby. The patient had, in fact, been correct about her time of conception, and the baby died from an expired placenta, poisoned by his own amniotic fluid. The lack of faith in a woman's understanding of her own body and no tests to accurately track pregnancy killed my uncle.

My grandmother was a devoted Catholic but since the baby had not yet been baptized, the church refused to allow my uncle to be buried in their cemetery. Not only did Grandma lose her son, but she also lost her faith and community, driving her pain and isolation even deeper.

In 1991 my mother was pregnant with me. And still, without fully understanding why contractions never started, Grandma reminded my pregnant mother that if she went past her due date, it was not because she had miscalculated, and no matter what, she needed to advocate for herself and her baby. Sure enough, I was two weeks past due and my mother petitioned for a C-section. When they extracted me from my mother's uterus, my legs were deformed. I became so large in the womb that my legs bent inwards, so my knees and toes faced each other. The first six weeks of my newborn life were spent in casts. Every week, my mother took her baby girl to the hospital for them to remove my casts, twist my legs, and reset them.

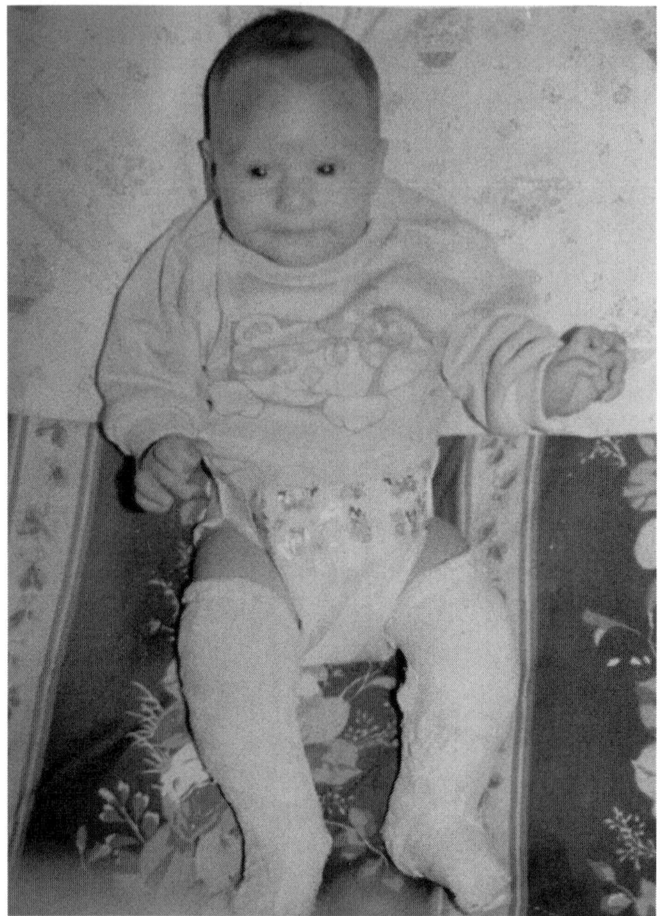

*Figure 1: Dr. Brittany Barreto at three months old and on her fifth set of leg casts to straighten her legs to walk one day successfully.*

Until age six, I wore medical boots with metal rods to straighten my feet—a small price to pay compared to my uncle.

My story is sadly not as uncommon as it should be. What we are realizing is that until recently, women's health has gone largely misunderstood, understudied, and neglected. As a result, women suffer not only in childbearing but also in menstruation, menopause, and postmenopause. Their physical, mental, emotional, spiritual, and financial health are all compromised in one way or another by the long history of underserved health needs.

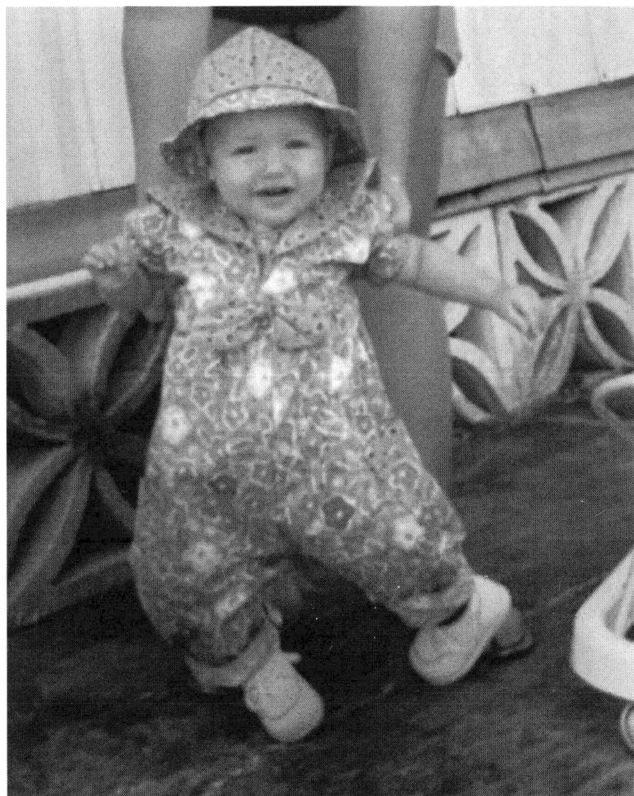

*Figure 2: Dr. Brittany Barreto, eleven months old, wearing shoes with metal siding to straighten her feet.*

Interestingly, women are well documented as intuiting when something is wrong within their bodies, an instinct that when voiced is often dismissed as being an overreaction, confusion, or attention-seeking behavior. The result is often disastrous, as shown in the story of my birth and the loss of my uncle.

What if we believed women about their bodies? What if we had medical devices and tests that accurately tracked pregnancy? Could we avoid these deaths and deformities? The women's health innovation movement, also known as FemTech, is here to do just that: to save lives and improve the health and wellness of everyone. When women's health is improved, so is everyone else's health, including men, communities, businesses, economies, and Mother Earth herself. Focusing on women's health is a turnkey solution to elevating all humanity.

## The State of Women's Health

The male bias in research and translational medicine has led to a healthcare system that, by design, favors male biology, leaving women's health needs and outcomes in the shadows. This systemic disparity is underscored by the staggering statistic that one-third of women in the United States undergoes a hysterectomy by the age of sixty, a testament to the medical community's default approach to treating women's health issues with drastic interventions rather than nuanced understanding and care. Between 1977 and 1993, women were outright banned from participating in clinical trials, meaning that no drug approved before this year had been tested on a woman of reproductive age.[1] This policy lapse contributed to the enduring knowledge gap in female biology and the efficacy of medical treatments on women.

The lack of focused research on conditions affecting women is exemplified by the National Institutes of Health (NIH) dedicating less than 0.00001 percent of its budget to menopause research in 2020, a field critical to understanding and improving the health of half the population as they age.[2] The use of male cell lines in 71 percent of scientific research further exacerbates the risk of misinterpreting data that may be male-specific, hindering the development of effective, sex-specific treatments.[3] Women, on average, spend nine years of their lives in poor health, which diminishes their presence and productivity in all facets of life, from home to the workforce, while also reducing their earning potential.[4]

Historically, the approach to women's health has been narrowly focused on reproductive capabilities—often dismissively dubbed "bikini medicine"—which mistakenly suggests that the primary differences between women and men are limited to menstruation, pregnancy, and breastfeeding. However, the FemTech sector boldly challenges this outdated notion with the assertion that women are *not* small men. This mis-conception has led to a profound gap in our understanding of sex-specific biological and pharmacological differences. Without a deep grasp of how sex influences biology at a molecular level, we cannot hope to address the significant healthcare disparities that affect those assigned female at birth —disparities that extend well beyond reproductive health.

The consequences of this gender disparity in healthcare are stark and quantifiable. Medicines are three and one-half times more likely to be withdrawn from the market for safety reasons affecting women than men, a clear indication of the healthcare innovation pipeline's failure to adequately consider female physiology. Furthermore, women in the United States report adverse events from approved medicines 52 percent more frequently than men, with serious or fatal events reported 36 percent more frequently. Diagnostic delays compound this problem. A study in Denmark found women are diagnosed later than men for over 700 diseases, with significant lags for conditions like cancer and diabetes.[5] In the United States, fewer than half of women living with endometriosis have a documented diagnosis, highlighting the pervasive underdiagnosis and undertreatment of women.[6] This male-centered paradigm in medicine has not only perpetuated a lack of knowledge about female biology but also has resulted in poorer health outcomes for women and a dire shortage of female-specific healthcare solutions.

## Introducing FemTech

In the landscape of technology-driven solutions for healthcare, FemTech emerges as a beacon of innovation, particularly addressing the unique health challenges and opportunities within the women's health sector. Coined by Ida Tin in 2016, founder of Clue, a period-tracking app, the term *FemTech* effectively bridges the gap between female health needs and technological advancements. Unlike generic searches for *women's health* that may lead to the address of a local WeightWatchers club, searching the term *FemTech* directs the inquirer toward cutting-edge technologies, investments, and innovations to enhance female health and wellness. This nomenclature has defined the sector and fostered a community, allowing stakeholders to find each other and collaborate under this unified banner. An industry that in 2019 had an unquantified market value, one venture fund, zero accelerators, and no community now has dozens of local and global organizations, eleven venture funds, and multiple accelerators. We could all identify with an industry that has since become a movement.

FemTech transcends the traditional confines of reproductive health, embracing a broader spectrum that includes conditions disproportionately or uniquely affecting females, women, and girls. From migraines and autoimmune diseases more prevalent in women to the sex-specific manifestations of conditions like breast cancer and heart disease, Fem-

Tech is at the forefront of addressing these disparities. Importantly, the industry acknowledges the intricate interplay between sex and gender and their impacts on health outcomes from conception. While biological sex can influence health directly, gender norms and roles significantly shape the perception, reporting, and treatment of conditions, often leading to gender bias in medical care. This bias manifests distinctly in the treatment of pain and chronic conditions, where women's experiences and symptoms are frequently underestimated or dismissed.

FemTech's inclusive approach extends to all who have been assigned female at birth and gender-identifying women, recognizing the unique health challenges faced by intersex, transmen, transwomen, and gender nonconforming individuals. The industry's commitment to inclusivity emphasizes the need for sex and gender considerations in research, diagnosis, and treatment across all ages, including young girls whose health needs are often generalized under children's health. As a female or a woman reading this book, you may not identify with every health challenge presented due to your own biology and anatomy because gender and sex are a spectrum and so too are the solutions created for these bodies and genders. As you read the words *female* and *woman* throughout this book, please know that this text is written from a core value of inclusivity.

The FemTech industry, a formidable market size of $1.2 trillion as of 2021, represents not just a sector within healthcare but a transformative movement redefining women's health and wellness.[7] This valuation, meticulously compiled from an analysis covering over 103 conditions across twenty-one health subsectors, starkly contrasts the previously under-estimated figure of $50 billion. The number discrepancy is not just a matter of arithmetic; it underscores a historical oversight in appreciating the full spectrum of women's health needs. Despite this groundbreaking revelation, significant areas within women's health remain unquantified, hinting at an even more expansive market potential. Notably, conditions like premenstrual syndrome (PMS) and procedures such as tubal ligation (referred to often as getting one's tubes tied) lack comprehensive market valuation, highlighting both the challenges and opportunities for future FemTech innovations.

The landscape of FemTech companies is as diverse as it is dynamic, spanning health verticals from gynecological care and menstruation to mental health and chronic conditions.

FEMHEALTH VERTICALS
ABORTION
BREAST HEALTH
BREAST FEEDING
CARDIOVASCULAR
CHRONIC CONDITIONS
CONTRACEPTION
FERTILITY
FITNESS
GENERAL HEALTH
HAIR
HORMONAL HEALTH
MATERNAL HEALTH
MENOPAUSE
MENSTRUATION
MENTAL HEALTH
OVARIAN HEALTH
PELVIC FLOOR HEALTH
REPRODUCTIVE HEALTH
SAFETY
SEXUAL WELLNESS
SKIN HEALTH
URINARY HEALTH
UTERINE HEALTH
VAGINAL HEALTH

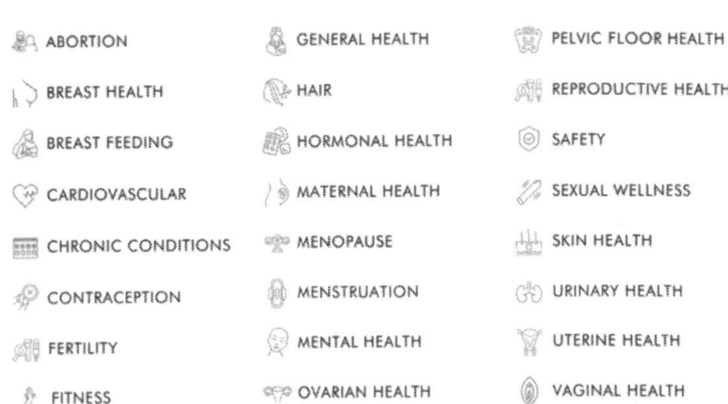

*Figure 3: FemTech innovates in a wide range of health and wellness verticals related to women's health.*[8]

As of Spring 2024, there are 1,416 active, global FemTech companies, with 50 percent founded in the last five years, signaling a robust growth trajectory.[9]

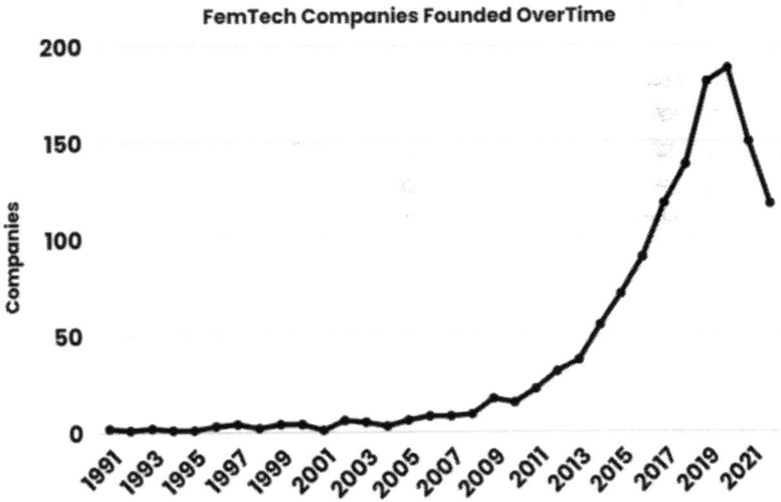


*Figure 4: FemTech companies founded over the last thirty years. The notable "drop" observed on the graph does not indicate a decline in the number of companies but rather reflects the methodology used to record them, which requires an active website for tracking. The number of startups founded between 2021 and 2023 is expected to climb to over 2,007.*

The proliferation of FemTech companies across product types—from digital health platforms and consumer packaged goods (CPG) to biotech assays and therapeutic drugs—reveals a multifaceted approach to women's health.

FEMHEALTH PRODUCT TYPES
APPAREL
BIOTECH
CONSUMER DIGITAL PRODUCT
CPG
DIAGNOSTICS
DIGITAL COMMUNITY
DIGITAL HEALTH
EDUCATIONAL PLATFORM
FINTECH
HEALTHCARE SOFTWARE
INSURTECH
LOGISITICS
MARKETPLACE
MEDICAL DEVICE
MEDICAL PROCEDURE
SUPPLEMENTS
TELEHEALTH
THERAPEUTIC DRUGS

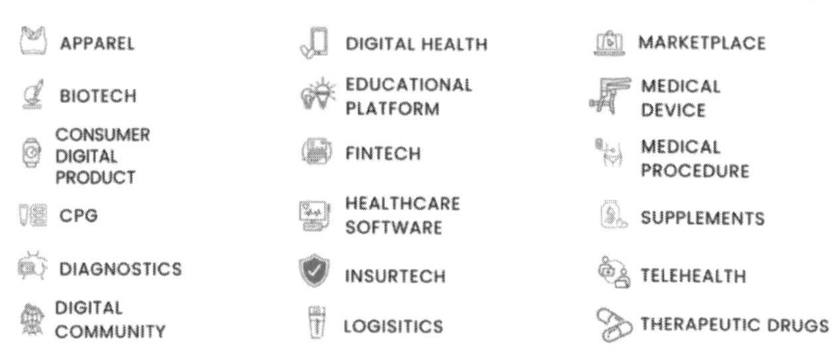

*Figure 5: FemTech innovation comes in a wide range of product types.*[10]

The surge in FemTech solutions is significantly influenced by the unique intersection of women's growing roles in finance, STEM, and the collective push toward destigmatizing female health. Remarkably, a study analyzing over 440,000 medical patents from 1976 to 2010 found that patents by female inventors were 35 percent more likely to benefit women's health, often targeting female-specific conditions like breast cancer and lupus.[11] Despite the historical underrepresentation of women in STEM, their presence in this sector has seen a commendable growth of 31 percent between 2011 and 2021, indicating a promising trend toward gender parity.[12] In the financial realm, while men continue to dominate, particularly in executive roles, the landscape is gradually shifting. Women now represent 42 percent of the finance sector workforce. Yet, a scant 32 percent ascend to executive positions, highlighting a disparity slowly being addressed as the industry acknowledges women's value in leadership roles.[13] The investment scene also reflects this positive trend, with only 5 percent of angel investors identifying as women in 2004 and by 2021 that percentage grew to 33.6 percent.[14] These shifts underscore a critical period of transformation where the integration of women into finance and STEM not only fosters gender diversity but also propels the development of innovative solutions addressing the unique health needs of women, paving the way for a more inclusive and equitable healthcare ecosystem.

We believe that FemTech is still in its earliest years of development and will continue to grow at a steady pace. The industry has already established itself as a legitime sector and not a fad.

Therefore, it is unsurprising that women overwhelmingly found FemTech companies. Today, 85 percent of FemTech companies have at least one female founder, higher than any other tech industry. This is truly an industry built and led *by* women, *for* women.[15]

While FemTech stands as a beacon of women's innovation and leadership, echoing our profound understanding and unique needs, its journey toward full potential is incomplete without the active participation of male allies. The essence of FemTech's success lies not only in female guidance—vital for its authenticity and relevance—but also in welcoming and embracing the support, insight, and collaboration of men who are equally passionate about revolutionizing women's health.

Some men have felt on the fringes of FemTech, perhaps confronting for the first time what it feels like to be a minority in a domain of innovation. This discomfort, while understandable, underscores a valuable shift in perspective, offering men a chance to engage in genuine partnership and equality. Numerous men in FemTech have already set a high bar, demonstrating that when we unite across gender lines with mutual respect and shared goals, we amplify our impact. Their dedication and insights enrich our mission, proving that FemTech's strength lies in diversity and inclusivity. I extend a warm invitation to more men to step into this transformative space, to contribute to and be part of creating a healthier future for women worldwide.

## What to Expect in This Book

In this book, readers are invited on an enlightening journey through the burgeoning field of FemTech, defined as solutions to conditions that solely, disproportionately, or differently affect females, women, and girls. Each chapter of the book serves as a gateway to one of fourteen crucial areas of women's health, ranging from puberty to dementia, unveiling the unique challenges and the evolving funding landscape that FemTech companies navigate. This book is designed to inform and showcase the breadth and depth of global innovations making strides in women's health.

Each chapter begins with an engaging introduction to a health vertical followed by excerpts from four to nine interviews per chapter, drawn from the *FemTech Focus* podcast—an initiative I launched in March 2020 amid the COVID-19 lockdown. Born from a profound need to fill the information void in the FemTech industry, the podcast has grown into a pivotal platform for dialogue and discovery, featuring over 250 episodes with insights from doctors, researchers, and innovators across the women's health spectrum. With 150,000 downloads and a reach spanning 148 countries as of spring 2024, the podcast has significantly contributed to demystifying and disseminating knowledge on FemTech. The featured, pioneering companies within each domain are not exhaustive in the least, but a small illumination of the incredible variety and scope of solutions being developed worldwide, highlighting the sector's vibrancy and the critical need for more visibility in these innovations. Listen to *FemTech Focus* podcasts to hear the full interviews of the innovators featured in this book and dozens more.

Through this text, readers will gain a comprehensive understanding of the disparities in healthcare and what FemTech entails and grasp the indispensable role of sex and gender in innovation. I aim for every reader to emerge as an advocate for FemTech, with the conviction that advancing women's health is fundamental to improving societal health for all. Let us champion the cause of FemTech in our daily lives, underscoring that women are not simply smaller men but individuals with unique health needs deserving of equitable healthcare solutions.

Health and wellness historically and presently are privileges where underserved demographics experience suboptimal solutions and worse outcomes. FemTech is more than a category of product types, it's a movement for equality in healthcare. That is why my deepest desire is that this book rapidly becomes outdated. I know you are the engineers, healthcare professionals, politicians, investors, teachers, advocates, scientists, entrepreneurs, researchers, students, and patients who will continue the movement and improve women's and female health. I hope this book becomes a historical context of what happens when diversity is not at the table and when we assume a single solution will work the same for everyone. May this text inspire you to lead a movement for equality and representation wherever there is injustice.

# Chapter 1
# Menstruation

**IN THE QUIET CONFINES OF THE MIDDLE SCHOOL BATHROOM,** Sarah discovered a stain of crimson on her pale-yellow dress—a stark contrast that sent waves of panic through her. She stood frozen, staring at her reflection, overwhelmed by embarrassment and confusion. Nobody had prepared her for this moment; discussions about adolescence had been abstract and veiled, leaving her to navigate this sudden reality alone. Hastily, she wrapped her sweater around her waist to conceal the stain and hurried out, her heart pounding with the fear of being discovered.

After school, Sarah's trip to the store felt like navigating an alien landscape, with aisles filled with products she hardly understood—pads, tampons, liners. Each glance from strangers felt like a spotlight on her vulnerability. Clutching her phone, she desperately searched online for guidance but only found her anxiety deepening with each unanswered question about the normalcy of her symptoms. At the shelves, a gentle woman noticed her distress and offered advice on selecting the right product for a beginner. Grateful for the kindness and feeling slightly relieved, Sarah left the store with a new sense of solidarity and understanding, armed with the essentials and the reassurance that she was not alone in her experience.

The act of menstruating is quite rare. Only 1.5 percent of all mammalian species on Earth have a menstrual cycle.[16] Besides primates, which include humans, apes, and old world and new world monkeys, the only other known species to menstruate are three species of bats and a family of rodents in Africa known as elephant shrews. Menstruation is something very special for humans.

Humans have periods because pregnancy is a very dangerous and energy-exhaustive experience. Due to the high risk of death from pregnancy and childbirth, the human body wants to be absolutely sure that the pregnancy is likely to be successful and safe. The period is a safety net in case the fetus is not viable. The female body can expel the endometrial lining (a period) along with any potential fertilized egg or fetus (miscarriage) that is unlikely to lead to a healthy baby. This is why we see 15 to 25 percent of fertilized eggs ending in miscarriage.[17]

Female humans spend an average of seven years bleeding throughout their lives.[18] That's over 300 periods between puberty and menopause. Females today have twice as many periods throughout their lives than any other females in history due to periods starting sooner for girls, increased life expectancy, and decreased number of pregnancies. Females do not have their periods during the nine months of gestation and typically do not have their periods during breastfeeding. Historically, females used to have upward of eight pregnancies and therefore had way fewer periods than the females of today with an average of two pregnancies.

Not only is menstruation challenged with being taboo in most cultures, but it also has environmental and public health challenges, such as the number of menstrual products going to landfills and the need for hygienic methods of washing nondisposable menstrual products. With a $43.25 billion global market size as of 2024 and over 32 percent of all FemTech products targeting menstruation, it is among the most innovative categories of women's health.[19,20] These innovations include cannabidiol, or CBD, in tampons to treat cramps, alternative materials to make pads sustainable, and new paradigms for how menstrual products are supplied.

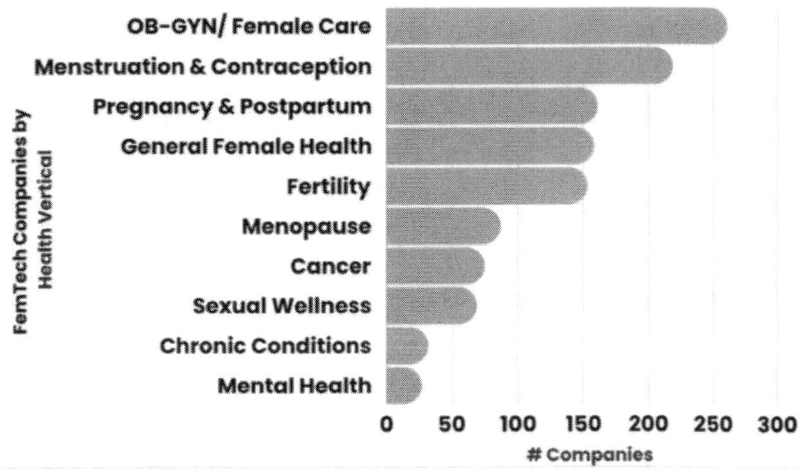


*Figure 6. Distribution of 1,416 women's health startups by health vertical that they are addressing.*[21]

Let's see how these innovators are addressing menstruation in a wide range of economies and through diverse ideas and strategies to make periods more comfortable, affordable, and safe.

## Milena Bacalja Perianes, Cofounder and Former Chief Research and Innovation Officer at Menstrual Health Hub

*Milena, a specialist in FemTech and gender lens investing, is dedicated to forging connections between the financial and social sectors to address gender health inequities. Her expertise in menstrual health comes from her prior venture, Menstrual Health Hub, a female health nonprofit and social impact business that fostered new investments in the menstrual health industry. Episode 23 aired June 23, 2020.*

### Why is there a need to consider women's experiences beyond just periods?

The menstrual cycle is one aspect of a much broader spectrum of women's health. When we consider menstrual health, we must think holistically about a woman's life and the various stages she goes through, including puberty, reproductive years, and menopause.

By understanding that a woman's body and health needs are continuously evolving, we can create menstrual products that are more than just functional; they can be supportive and adaptable to these changes. For instance, the design of menstrual products can be improved to cater to different life stages, such as postpartum or perimenopausal needs, where a woman's body undergoes significant changes.

Moreover, it's not just about the physical aspect of menstruation. We need to address the social and emotional dimensions of menstrual health. This includes tackling the stigma and misinformation surrounding menstruation and promoting open and inclusive conversations about it. By doing so, we can develop products that are both physically comfortable and suitable and empower women to feel confident and dignified during their menstrual cycle.

Innovation in menstrual products should also consider environmental sustainability and cultural sensitivity. Considering the significant waste generated by menstrual products each year, we need environmentally friendly as well as culturally sensitive products that respect and adapt to different cultural norms and practices around menstruation.

## What's the current state of menstrual wellness?

The current state of global menstrual wellness is a complex picture with progress and ongoing challenges. On the positive side, we have seen significant strides in awareness and breaking down taboos surrounding menstruation. More countries and organizations acknowledge menstrual health as a critical aspect of women's health and rights. There are increasing initiatives, both at grassroots and policy levels, to improve menstrual health education, and increase access to menstrual products and sanitary facilities.

However, challenges remain substantial. Globally, there are still millions of women and girls who lack access to safe, affordable menstrual products. This lack of access is not confined to developing countries; it's also a concern in developed nations, where issues like period poverty affect marginalized communities the most. Inadequate menstrual hygiene directly impacts education, livelihoods, and overall quality of life as girls often miss school, work, and community activities during their periods.

Another critical challenge is the persistent stigma and myths surrounding menstruation. In many cultures, menstruation is still shrouded in secrecy and shame, leading to misinformation and a lack of open conversation about menstrual health. This stigma can have profound implications on mental health and social inclusion.

From a medical perspective, there's still a lack of comprehensive research on menstrual disorders such as endometriosis, polycystic ovary syndrome (PCOS), and premenstrual syndrome (PMS), which affects a significant number of women. Diagnosis and treatment of these conditions often come with challenges due to limited understanding and awareness.

Looking forward, we need a more holistic approach to menstrual wellness encompassing education, access to menstrual products, safe sanitation facilities, and to break down cultural taboos. It's also crucial to integrate menstrual health into broader health and education policies to ensure that the needs of all menstruating individuals are met. Collaborative efforts among governments, NGOs, healthcare providers, educators, and communities are essential to make menstrual wellness a global priority. But women do not always have access to the products they need, let alone the ones they prefer.

## Claire Coder, Founder and CEO at Aunt Flow

*Aunt Flow offers a range of dispensing systems for tampons and pads and touch-free disposal units, primarily for use in public and private facilities. Episode 133 aired September 13, 2021.*

### Tell us about menstrual products in public bathrooms and how it's changing.

We're witnessing a remarkable transformation in the availability of menstrual products in public restrooms, particularly in educational settings. This shift is both a reflection of and a catalyst for broader societal changes in how we approach menstruation.

Let's look at the legislative landscape in the US as an example. In 2014, no states had mandates to provide free menstrual products in middle and high school bathrooms. Fast forward to 2020, and twenty-four states have taken the significant step of requiring these products in at least 50 percent of school bathrooms. This legislation progression highlights the issue and ensures that menstrual products are accessible in a dignified way, thus eliminating the often embarrassing and impractical need for students to visit the nurse's office for these essentials.

But what's even more compelling is this change's impact on student attendance. At Aunt Flow, we've found that schools offering free menstrual products see a 2.4 percent increase in attendance among female students.[22] This statistic is eye-opening and underscores the prevalence of period poverty right here in the US. It's not just a global issue; it's affecting students in our own backyard, hindering their education due to a lack of basic necessities.

The push for these changes often comes from the students themselves, showcasing the power and determination of young activists. These students are advocating for themselves and playing a critical role in transforming the entire educational system to be more inclusive and equitable.

When we talk about providing free menstrual products in public restrooms, it's not just about convenience or health. It's about educational equity and ensuring that every student can attend school without the barrier of menstrual inequity. The impact of these initiatives goes beyond just improving access; it's about changing lives and creating opportunities for students who were previously held back due to a lack of resources.

This is why the work we do at Aunt Flow is so crucial, and it's why we'll continue to push for changes that make menstrual products as commonplace and accessible as toilet paper in every restroom. It's not just a matter of comfort; it's a matter of basic human rights and dignity.

### What's the problem with coin-operated product dispensers?

To start, they need to be updated and more reliable. How often have you or someone you know needed a tampon or pad, and found a coin-operated dispenser, only to realize it's either empty or broken? Plus, the very idea that you need to pay for something as essential as menstrual products is frankly archaic. It's like having to insert a quarter for toilet paper—it just doesn't make sense.

And then there are the logistics of managing the coins collected from these dispensers; it is a headache for facilities. Someone must count the money, take it to the bank, and ensure it is properly accounted for. It's an inefficient system that creates unnecessary complexity and cost.

At Aunt Flow, we decided to tackle this problem head-on. We've created a range of free-vend tampon and pad dispensers that eliminate the need for coins altogether. Our dispensers are not only more user-friendly but also more dignified. We believe that access to menstrual products is a right, not a privilege, so we designed our dispensers to be as accessible as possible.

Our dispensers come in several models to fit different needs. They're easy to use, easy to restock, and don't require payment or coins, so anyone who needs a product can get one without hassle. We've also focused on making them ADA-compliant, with features like braille and easy-to-push buttons. At our company, we polled many users to make sure we maintained our focus on inclusivity and ensured that these products are accessible to all who need them.

This shift to free-vend dispensers is changing the landscape in restrooms. It's about changing the narrative around menstrual equity and accessibility. We're seeing businesses, schools, and other organizations recognizing the importance of providing menstrual products as a necessity. It's a shift toward recognizing menstruation as a standard, natural part of life that shouldn't be hidden away or treated as an inconvenience. By making menstrual products freely accessible, we're not just providing a service but a statement about the importance of menstrual equity and dignity. And that includes how the menstrual cycle affects our everyday lives from exercise to productivity.

## Hélène Guillaume Pabis, Founder and CEO at Wild.AI

*Wild.AI is at the forefront of integrating the menstrual cycle into women's fitness and health routines. Women can optimize their performance and overall well-being by offering personalized training plans and nutrition recommendations aligned with the menstrual cycle.*
*Episode 49 aired September 28, 2020.*

### Why should female athletes track their periods?

A critical issue in women's health that's often overlooked is amenorrhea (loss of period), especially in athletes. It's a misconception that losing one's period is a normal consequence of high-level athletic training. This is far from the truth. It's often a sign of nutritional imbalances, leading to serious concerns like reduced bone density and increased risk of osteoporosis, particularly postmenopause.

For several reasons, understanding and tracking the menstrual cycle is crucial for female athletes. First, the menstrual cycle significantly impacts an athlete's physiology, affecting everything from energy levels to injury risk. For instance, hormonal fluctuations can influence joint laxity, making injuries like ACL tears more likely during certain cycle phases. Tracking their cycles allows athletes to adapt their training to mitigate these risks.

Training with the menstrual cycle in mind is not just about avoiding injuries, it's also about optimizing performance. Different cycle phases can affect an athlete's strength, endurance, and recovery times. For example, some women may have more strength and endurance during the follicular phase after menstruation due to lower progesterone levels. By aligning training with these physiological changes, athletes can maximize their performance and recovery.

Historically, women haven't incorporated their menstrual cycle into their athletic training largely due to a lack of awareness and research. Menstruation and the menstrual cycle have been taboo topics, often not openly discussed, even in athletic circles. Additionally, much of the existing sports science research has been based on male athletes and assumes that findings apply equally to women. This gender bias in research has led to a significant knowledge gap regarding the unique physiological needs of female athletes.

Moreover, there's been a pervasive myth that a woman's period is a hindrance to her athletic performance. This myth, coupled with the lack of tailored guidance for female athletes, has led to a one-size-fits-all approach to training, which often ignores the menstrual cycle's impact.

However, the tide is turning. There's growing recognition of the importance of sex-specific research in sports science. More female athletes are speaking out about their experiences and advocating for a more informed approach to training that considers the menstrual cycle. Apps and technologies are emerging to help track and integrate these insights into training programs. It's a crucial step toward personalized, effective training for female athletes, enabling them to train smarter, not just harder.

## How does Wild.AI incorporate the female menstrual cycle?

Only in July 2019 did Apple introduce a period-tracking feature in its Health app. This was a significant step, albeit late, considering the substantial portion of women in their user base. It's reflective of a broader trend where women's health needs are often an afterthought in technology—something we're actively working to change.

Wild.AI is a revolutionary platform specifically designed for female athletes. It recognizes the unique physiological and hormonal variations that women experience. Our primary goal is to empower female athletes by providing them with personalized insights and guidance that align with their menstrual cycles.

What sets Wild.AI apart is its holistic approach to training, nutrition, and recovery. We understand that a woman's body is not static; it changes throughout the menstrual cycle. Our app tracks these changes and adjusts recommendations accordingly. For example, when estrogen levels are higher during the follicular phase, and women generally feel stronger, our app might suggest more intense training sessions. Conversely, when some women feel more fatigued during the luteal phase, the app might recommend lighter workouts and focus on recovery.

Wild.AI also strongly emphasizes nutrition. We recognize that nutritional needs fluctuate throughout the menstrual cycle. The app provides tailored dietary suggestions to optimize performance and health, whether recommending more iron-rich foods during menstruation or adjusting carbohydrate intake during different cycle phases.

Recovery is another crucial aspect. The app suggests specific recovery techniques based on the menstrual cycle phase, helping athletes avoid overtraining and reduce the risk of injuries. For instance, it will suggest low-impact exercises and additional muscle-strengthening workouts during increased joint laxity to prevent injuries like ACL tears.

Moreover, Wild.AI is more than just an app; it's a platform for research and education. We're committed to advancing the understanding of female physiology in sports. We aim to fill the knowledge gap in women's sports science by collecting data and sharing insights. We're proud to be among FemTech companies that are challenging the status quo of what we perceive as normal for periods—even things we did not think we could control, like menstrual pain.

## Valentina Milanova, Founder and CEO at Daye

*Daye's innovative pain-relieving, CBD-infused organic tampons, featuring a biobased applicator and a water-soluble wrapper for convenient disposal are pushing boundaries in menstrual product innovation.*
*Episode 105 aired April 11, 2021.*

### What is the history of how women's menstrual pain has been perceived?

Throughout history, menstrual pain has often been trivialized and overlooked, a pattern that unfortunately persists in many parts of the world. For a long time, and regrettably still in some cases, menstrual pain hasn't been given the medical attention it deserves. Historically, women's health issues, including menstrual pain, have been sidelined in medical research and discussion. It's been a struggle to get menstrual pain recognized as a legitimate medical issue, rather than just a part of being a woman.

One striking example is the story of Viagra, which sheds light on the skewed priorities in medical research. Viagra, now known for treating erectile dysfunction, was initially explored as a medication for menstrual pain. However, despite presenting two research proposals to the National Institutes of Health, one focusing on Viagra's potential for relieving menstrual pain and the other on erectile dysfunction, the NIH chose to fund the latter. This decision was made even though menstrual pain affects a staggering 90 percent of women, while erectile dysfunction affects only about 19 percent of men. It's a clear illustration of how women's health issues, particularly those as common as menstrual pain, have been historically undervalued and under-researched.

This pattern of sidelining women's health is further exemplified by the case of Procter & Gamble in the 1980s. They considered developing a pain-relieving tampon but ultimately scrapped the idea, believing the market was too small. This decision underscores a persistent underestimation of the impact of menstrual pain on women's lives.

Another example is the use of common painkillers like Advil. For years, women have been using pain relief medication that was formulated based on male physiology. It's only recently that the recommended dosage of painkillers like ibuprofen for women has been reevaluated. Women often need a higher dosage, 800 milligrams compared to the standard 250 milligrams, to effectively manage menstrual pain. This discrepancy in dosage is a direct result of the historical exclusion of women from clinical drug trials until as recently as 1993. The effect of this exclusion has been a widespread lack of understanding and adequate treatment for women's specific health needs, particularly concerning menstrual pain.

In more recent times, there's been a gradual shift toward acknowledging and addressing menstrual pain. However, the journey is far from over. There's still a considerable gap in understanding and addressing menstrual pain effectively. Women's experiences with menstrual pain are diverse, and there's a pressing need for more research and solutions that cater specifically to women's needs. For too long, women have had to endure menstrual pain silently, but it's high time that this changes. We must continue pushing for more awareness, research, and solutions tailored to women's unique health needs.

## What has Daye created? How can cannabinoids be uniquely useful for period pain?

Daye has taken a novel approach to menstrual care by creating a tampon that not only meets the highest standards of safety and sustainability but also addresses the often-overlooked issue of period pain. Our product is a culmination of rigorous research and innovation, particularly focusing on the use of cannabinoids for menstrual pain relief.

Cannabinoids, particularly CBD (cannabidiol), have unique properties that make them highly effective for managing period pain. Unlike traditional painkillers, which can have a delayed onset and various side effects, cannabinoids provide a more natural and targeted approach to pain relief. CBD has anti-inflammatory and analgesic properties, which are crucial in alleviating the discomfort caused by menstrual cramps. When used in a tampon, CBD can be delivered directly to the source of pain, offering faster and more efficient relief compared to oral medications.

Daye's tampons are designed with a protective sleeve to prevent fiber shedding and are sterilized using a safe gamma ray process, ensuring they are free from bacteria and pathogens. This level of attention to safety and hygiene is something we take very seriously.

Furthermore, the environmental impact of menstrual products is a growing concern. At Daye, we address this by using sustainable materials like biodegradable sugarcane for our applicators and water-soluble wrappers. This reflects our commitment not only to women's health but also to the health of our planet.

At Daye, we've gone beyond the traditional approach to menstrual care by focusing on pain relief and prioritizing the highest standards of hygiene and safety in our tampons. An aspect that distinctly sets us apart is our commitment to sterilization of the tampons after manufacturing and before being sold, a step that is surprisingly not mandated by government regulations for tampon manufacturing. This is startling, considering that tampons are inserted into one of the most absorbent and sensitive parts of the female body. Recognizing this gap in safety standards, Daye has proactively implemented a sterilization process in our manufacturing. However, many aspects of menstrual-product design and production have not taken into account the safety of women or the environment.

## Olivia Ahn, MBBS, Cofounder at Planera

*Planera.care addresses the environmental impact of disposable menstrual products with 100 percent flushable and biodegradable sanitary pads. Episode 91 aired February 19, 2021.*

### What is the environmental impact of menstrual products?

The environmental impact of menstrual products is a significant and often-overlooked issue. Traditional menstrual products like pads and tampons contribute enormously to environmental pollution. For instance, in the UK alone, it's estimated that over 200,000 tons of menstrual waste is generated annually, equivalent to around 17,000 London buses. This waste predominantly ends up in landfills, taking up to 500 years to degrade due to the high plastic content, and nearly 90 percent of every tampon is plastic.

Moreover, about 30 percent of these products end up in waterways, causing blockages and contributing to marine pollution. These figures are staggering when they represent just one small, island nation. Expanding this globally, the volume of menstrual waste is enough to wrap around the Earth multiple times.

The main problem lies in the design of these products. They contain plastics in the adhesive, the backing sheet, and the super absorbent polymers. Even products labeled as organic only replace the top sheet with cotton, leaving the rest of the plastic components intact. This is why at Planera, we're focusing on creating not only biodegradable but also flushable products, aligning with existing sewage infrastructure and offering a more environmentally friendly disposal method.

### What is Planera and how are your products innovative?

Planera is a personal hygiene company, and our mission is rooted in the belief that disposable, consumable products need to be rethought regarding their disposal and environmental impact. Our first and flagship product is a 100 percent certified, flushable, and biodegradable sanitary pad. This innovation addresses a significant environmental challenge: the disposal of menstrual products.

Traditional sanitary products, such as pads and tampons, have a substantial environmental footprint. They typically contain plastic and other nonbiodegradable materials, contributing to landfill waste and waterway pollution. In contrast, our pads are designed to be flushed safely, breaking down just like toilet paper in the sewage system. This eliminates the need for landfill space and reduces the potential for waterway pollution.

Our pads are unique because they are made using advanced materials and a novel manufacturing process. Unlike traditional pads which use plastic components, our pads are crafted from plant-based cellulose fibers, making them biodegradable. Additionally, we've developed a process that doesn't rely on the usual thermoplastic materials; instead, we use a friction-based method to bind the layers of the pad, further reducing the environmental impact.

This innovation in menstrual care is a leap toward a more sustainable future, demonstrating that it's possible to create products that are effective and comfortable for the user and also kind to the planet. At Planera, we're committed to continuing our journey of innovating and improving personal hygiene products, making them sustainable and accessible to everyone because we need to take care of Mother Earth as much as she takes care of us.

## Kate Morton, MS, RDN, Founder and CEO at Funk It Wellness

*Funk It Wellness introduces the concept of seed cycling, emphasizing the role of nutrition in balancing hormones throughout the menstrual cycle. Seed cycling a simple and effective method that involves tracking your menstrual cycle and incorporating specific seeds into your diet at different times of the month. Episode 122 aired June 27, 2021.*

### What are the nutritional needs of a female throughout her menstrual cycle?

The female menstrual cycle is a complex and fascinating process, and nutrition is critical in supporting it. A cycle is divided into four phases: menstrual, follicular, ovulation, and luteal. Each phase has unique hormonal changes and different nutritional needs.

During the menstrual phase, our bodies experience inflammation as they shed the uterine lining. Nutrients like magnesium and omega-3s in pumpkin and flax seeds are incredibly helpful here. Magnesium aids in mood-boosting, while omega-3s assist in reducing inflammation and promoting estrogen detoxification.

As we move into the follicular phase, leading up to ovulation, our bodies prepare for the potential of pregnancy. A rise in energy and creativity characterizes this phase. Nutritional support during this phase focuses on zinc and magnesium to continue supporting mood and hormonal balance.

Ovulation is the peak of the cycle. It's when we're most fertile, and many women feel their best: energetic and vibrant. Vitamin E, found in sesame and sunflower seeds, is particularly beneficial during this phase. It helps with breast tenderness and continues to support overall hormonal health.

Finally, the luteal phase is when our bodies prepare for pregnancy or the next menstrual cycle. This phase can often bring PMS symptoms. Eating a diet rich in manganese and magnesium during this phase can help alleviate some of these symptoms.

## What is seed cycling and how can it support women throughout their menstrual cycle?

Seed cycling is a fascinating and natural approach to supporting hormonal balance throughout a woman's menstrual cycle. It involves consuming specific seeds during different phases of the cycle to provide targeted, nutritional support. The concept is rooted in the idea that certain seeds can help modulate hormone levels, alleviating menstrual symptoms and promoting overall hormonal health.

During the first phase (the menstrual phase) and the follicular phase leading up to ovulation, consuming flax and pumpkin seeds is beneficial. These seeds are rich in omega-3 fatty acids and lignans, which help manage estrogen levels and reduce inflammation. They're also high in magnesium, which is excellent for mood-boosting and alleviating menstrual cramps.

As we transition into the ovulation and luteal phases, the focus shifts to sesame and sunflower seeds. These seeds are packed with selenium and vitamin E, key for progesterone support. Vitamin E is particularly helpful in reducing breast tenderness, a common premenstrual symptom. The seeds also contain zinc and manganese, supporting hormonal balance and reducing PMS symptoms.

The beauty of seed cycling is that it aligns with the body's natural rhythm. By consuming these seeds, we provide our bodies with the nutrients they need to support each cycle phase. It's about empowering our bodies through nutrition, in a way that's aligned with our natural processes. Plus, it's a simple and delicious addition to your diet; you can sprinkle these ground seeds on salads, blend them into smoothies, or even include them in energy balls.

What I love about seed cycling is the potential physical benefits and the mindset it fosters. It encourages us to tune into our bodies, understand our cycles better, and take a proactive role in our health. It's a holistic approach, emphasizing the connection between what we eat and how we feel throughout our menstrual cycle.

Funk It Wellness provides the prepackaged and ground seeds conveniently delivered to your door. Each delivery has two bags of seeds. The first is for days one (period) through fourteen (typically, day fourteen denotes ovulation), and the second is for days fifteen (ovulation) through twenty-eight (last day before period returns). It's as easy as choosing the appropriate bag for your current menstrual phase and consuming two tablespoons of seeds daily. We have many yummy recipes and ways to easily incorporate seeds into your diet on our website and social channels. We are even launching product lines for other hormonal fluctuations in a woman's life such as entering menopause or experiencing low sexual libido. Using seeds and nutrition to optimize the menstrual cycle and decrease symptoms can elevate a woman's entire lifestyle including her productivity.

## Alyx Coble-Frakes, Founder and CEO at The Agenda

*The Agenda app is revolutionizing productivity by aligning tasks and activities with the four phases of the menstrual cycle. This innovative tool recognizes the impact of hormonal fluctuations on energy levels and creativity, enabling women to optimize their work and personal lives accordingly. Episode 126 aired July 29, 2021.*

### How does the menstrual cycle affect productivity?

The menstrual cycle profoundly impacts productivity, and aligning work tasks with each phase can significantly boost efficiency and well-being. Let's break down the cycle into four phases: menstrual, follicular, ovulation, and luteal.

During the menstrual phase, which is similar to winter, there's a natural tendency to turn inward and reflect. It's a period of higher intuition, where the left and right brain hemispheres communicate effectively. This is an ideal time for planning and strategizing rather than engaging in high-energy tasks.

Moving into the follicular phase, which I liken to spring, there's a surge in energy levels. Estrogen and follicle-stimulating hormones are rising, making it a fantastic time for active, engaging tasks like networking and initiating new projects. It's about putting the plan into action.

The ovulation phase is the powerhouse for communication and magnetism, much like the summer. It's the shortest phase, but during this time, our ability to articulate ideas and influence others is at its peak. This is the perfect time for important meetings, sales pitches, or asking for a raise.

Finally, the luteal phase, our autumn, is the longest and most complex. It starts with a burst of energy, ideal for critical decision-making and wrapping up projects; think of it as a harvest period. As the phase progresses, it's time to slow down, evaluate, and prepare for the next cycle.

Understanding and harnessing these phases can lead to more productive and fulfilling work experiences. It's about aligning with our natural rhythms, rather than fighting against them.

### What is the economic burden of not structuring work around the female hormone cycle?

The economic burden of ignoring the female hormone cycle in the workplace is substantial, impacting both productivity and absenteeism. A key study showed that not supporting women in the workforce with their menstrual health concerns leads to approximately nine days of lost productivity per year. This is a combination of reduced presenteeism, where women are at work but not fully functioning due to menstrual symptoms, and absenteeism, where they have to take time off.

To put this into perspective, consider the financial impact. If we multiply the number of women in the workforce by the average hourly wage, the loss to the economy is staggering. In the US alone, this can translate to billions of dollars annually. This isn't just a health issue; it's a significant economic concern.

Beyond the direct financial implications, there's also the issue of workplace morale and employee satisfaction. Women who feel unsupported in managing their menstrual health will likely be less engaged and may seek employment elsewhere. This turnover leads to additional recruitment and training costs for businesses.

The solution is recognizing and accommodating the natural fluctuations in women's productivity across their menstrual cycle. By doing so, we support the well-being of half the workforce and optimize their contributions, leading to a healthier, more productive, and economically robust working environment. Menstruators can bio-hack themselves into their best, happiest, most productive selves if they can track their cycle accurately and consistently and then plan around their hormone cycle.

* * *

In conclusion, menstruation, a natural yet complex phenomenon, represents a pivotal aspect of women's health and a significant opportunity for innovation and progress within the FemTech industry. From its rare biological occurrence to its profound impact on women's daily lives and societal participation, understanding menstruation goes beyond the biological narrative to encompass environmental, technological, and socio-economic dimensions. Innovations like CBD-infused tampons, flushable sanitary pads, and apps that align productivity with the menstrual cycle are just the beginning of a much-needed revolution in menstrual health and wellness. As we advance, it's crucial to continue breaking taboos, fostering inclusive discussions, and championing innovations that honor the unique needs of menstruators across the globe. The journey toward a more informed, empathetic, and sustainable approach to menstruation is not just about creating better products; it's about reshaping perceptions, policies, and practices to uplift and empower not only everyone who has or will menstruate but also those who are raising or impacting those who will one day menstruate.

# Chapter 2
# Uterine Health

**FOR TWENTY DAYS, AMANI HAD BEEN TRAPPED** in a relentless cycle of pain and exhaustion, each day bleeding as heavily as the last. In her family, stories of "strong women enduring strong periods" were passed down like heirlooms. Amani clung to this narrative, convincing herself that her experience was nothing unusual. Yet, as the days stretched, a nagging doubt began to take root in her mind. How long was too long? How much was too much? These questions circled endlessly, unanswered. But life, with its myriad demands, left little room for contemplation. As a single mother juggling a full-time job, the thought of taking time off to visit an OB-GYN—two hours away—seemed as feasible as a distant dream. Childcare was another puzzle with no solution in sight. And so, Amani endured, telling herself that this was simply the lot of the women in her family.

Amani's relationship with healthcare had always been fraught with tension and disbelief. Dismissive comments about her weight marred past visits to the OB-GYN, each appointment leaving her feeling more invisible, more unheard. It was as if her symptoms were mere whispers against a backdrop of preconceived notions. The idea of stepping into another clinic, only to have her pain attributed to her weight or dismissed altogether, was a battle she wasn't sure she had the strength to fight. Yet, in the quiet moments between her responsibilities, a darker fear whispered to her—the specter of uterine cancer, a disease that had claimed her grandmother. Amani would quickly shove these thoughts aside, refusing to entertain them. Cancer was a reality too harsh, too final for her already burdened shoulders to bear.

The uterus, also known as the womb, is a key player in women's health and reproductive systems. It's a pear-shaped organ, located deep in the pelvis, approximately the size of an orange. It plays a critical role in nurturing the fertilized ovum which then develops into a fetus. However, despite its vital function, uterine health is often shrouded in mystery and misunderstanding, leading to numerous health challenges for women globally.

The uterus is a dynamic organ held within the pelvis by several ligaments. It consists of three main sections: the fundus, the main body, and the cervix. The inner lining of the uterus, known as the endometrium, plays a crucial role during menstruation and pregnancy.

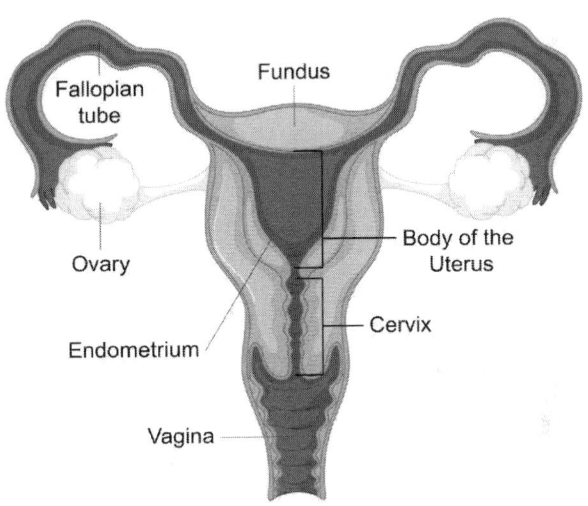


*Illustration showing the female reproductive system, and the sections of the uterus.*

*Figure 7: Diagram of the female reproductive system including the uterus, cervix, fallopian tubes, and ovaries.*

Uterine health is susceptible to various conditions, significantly impacting women's quality of life and the economy. Among these, endometriosis, adenomyosis, uterine fibroids, and uterine cancer are the most prevalent. To address them, we need to clearly understand what they are and how many are affected.

Endometriosis: Affecting roughly 10 percent of reproductive-age women globally, endometriosis occurs when tissue similar to the uterine lining grows outside the uterus, causing severe pain, heavy bleeding, and potential fertility issues.[23] Its diagnosis is often complicated, leading to delays in effective treatment. Environmental factors, such as exposure to certain chemicals and pesticides, have been linked to an increased risk of developing endometriosis.[24]

Adenomyosis: This condition involves the growth of endometrial tissue into the uterine muscle, leading to heavy periods, severe cramping, and an enlarged uterus. It affects approximately 20 percent of menstruators and is often managed through pain medications, hormonal treatments, and, in severe cases, hysterectomy.[25]

Uterine Fibroids: In 20-70 percent of women during their reproductive years, fibroids are noncancerous growths that can vary in size and number. While many women with fibroids are asymptomatic, others may experience heavy bleeding, pelvic pain, and reproductive complications.[26] Treatment options range from medication to surgical interventions.

Uterine Cancer: As a significant health concern, uterine cancer requires early detection and treatment. Its symptoms include abnormal vaginal bleeding, pelvic pain, and changes in menstrual cycles. Approximately 13,250 women die each year in the United States and 97,370 globally due to uterine cancer.[27,28]

Uterine health conditions affect individual women and have a broader economic impact. The cost of treating conditions like endometriosis, for instance, includes healthcare expenses, loss of productivity, and a diminished quality of life. Moreover, these conditions can affect mental health, relationships, and career progression. Employers are also beginning to recognize the importance of supporting women's health, as addressing these conditions can reduce absenteeism and enhance overall well-being in the workforce.

The history of uterine conditions such as endometriosis is a tale of misconceptions, struggles, and gradual scientific enlightenment that spans over 4,000 years. It was initially described in medical literature nearly 300 years ago, but its earliest mention dates back to Ancient Egypt's Ebers Papyrus around 1550 BC.[29] However, for centuries, the debilitating pain associated with endometriosis was misunderstood, and often dismissed as hysteria or a product of immorality.

During the Middle Ages, women experiencing severe pelvic pain were often labeled as mad or immoral, their symptoms attributed to their mental state rather than a physical ailment.[30] This perspective persisted for centuries, as the term *hysteria*, derived from the Latin word for womb (*hystericus*) became synonymous with exaggerated emotions and was linked to women's reproductive health.

The condition was misdiagnosed and mistreated for millennia, with treatments ranging from leeches to genital mutilation and exorcism. In the modern era, endometriosis is still frequently misunderstood, with many women normalizing their pain or encountering dismissive attitudes from healthcare professionals. This has led to a significant delay in diagnosis, averaging seven to ten years, and has often resulted in inappropriate treatments, including early hysterectomies or oophorectomies.[31]

However, the past few centuries have seen significant advancements. In the mid-1800s, pathologist Karl Freiherr von Rokitansky described the condition, marking a pivotal moment in its medical recognition.[32] Throughout the twentieth century, endometriosis began to be more accurately understood and diagnosed, thanks in part to developments in minimally invasive surgical procedures and a growing understanding of its genetic and immune components.

Despite these advancements, the historical stigma around endometriosis has persisted, with the condition often trivialized or overlooked in medical training. Medical gaslighting occurs when healthcare professionals minimize or dismiss patients' symptoms, suggesting that their experiences are imagined or exaggerated, rather than acknowledging them as legitimate medical concerns. This form of systemic dismissiveness has particularly profound impacts on women, who are affected by conditions like uterine fibroids, endometriosis, and uterine cancer. The journey to a correct diagnosis can be agonizingly prolonged, often spanning years, during which women are forced to navigate a labyrinth of skepticism and disbelief. This invalidation not only exacerbates their physical suffering but also inflicts deep psychological wounds, eroding their trust in the medical system and their own perceptions of reality. The emotional toll is compounded by the potential consequences of delayed diagnosis, such as chronic pain, severe menstrual bleeding, and infertility, which can profoundly affect a woman's quality of life and mental health. The struggle extends beyond the physical symptoms to a fight for recognition, understanding, and appropriate medical care, highlighting a critical need for systemic change within the healthcare industry to better listen to and validate women's health experiences.

Only recently, driven by patient advocacy and global awareness campaigns, has endometriosis started to gain the attention it requires as a serious, full-body disease. This shift is reflected in national action plans, increased research output, and the establishment of support groups.

The future of uterine health is promising but requires continued attention and investment. Research gaps must be addressed, particularly in understanding how lifestyle, nutrition, medications, and chronic conditions affect uterine health. Personalized medicine approaches should be prioritized to provide tailored advice and treatment for women with unique health profiles.

The efforts of these innovative organizations and individuals in uterine health are changing the landscape for women. With advancements in diagnostics, treatment options, advocacy, and awareness, we are moving closer to a future where these conditions are better understood, and more effectively managed, and the quality of life for those affected is significantly improved.

## Somer Baburek, MBA, Cofounder and CEO at Hera Biotech

*Hera Biotech is developing and commercializing the first nonsurgical, tissue-based test for the definitive diagnosis and staging of endometriosis. Episode 112 aired on May 3, 2021.*

### What is endometriosis?

Endometriosis is a condition where the tissue similar to the lining inside the uterus, called the endometrium, starts growing outside the uterus. This tissue can be found anywhere in the abdomen, and its growth can lead to severe pain, inflammation, and even pelvic adhesions. It's also the number one cause of female infertility. The exact cause of endometriosis is still not fully understood. Still, it's believed to be linked to genetic factors, particularly the dysregulation of certain genes responsible for cell adhesion and communication, like connexins.

Currently, the only definitive way to diagnose endometriosis is through a surgical procedure, specifically laparoscopic surgery. This involves inserting instruments into the abdomen to look for and biopsy suspected tissue. However, this method is invasive and not always conclusive. Additionally, there's no direct treatment for endometriosis itself; the available treatments are more focused on managing symptoms. These include drugs for pain management, hormonal therapies to suppress estrogen (since endometriosis is estrogen-driven), and in extreme cases, surgeries like hysterectomies are performed.

What's crucial to understand is that early diagnosis is key to managing endometriosis effectively. Despite the lack of a direct cure, knowing about the condition early on can help a person make informed decisions about treatments and managing symptoms, improving the quality of life.

## What is Hera Biotech creating?

Hera Biotech is creating the first nonsurgical, definitive diagnostic test for endometriosis that can also stage the disease. This is significant because currently, the only way to diagnose endometriosis is through invasive laparoscopic surgery, which is not only a challenging procedure but also often inconclusive for diagnosing the condition.

Our test is based on a deep understanding of the genetics and cellular behavior associated with endometriosis. We've identified specific genetic markers dysregulated in women with endometriosis, particularly those related to cell adhesion and communication. By analyzing these markers, our test can confirm the presence of endometriosis and determine the disease's stage.

The impact of this diagnostic test will be substantial. Early and accurate diagnosis of endometriosis can lead to better management of the condition, potentially improving the quality of life for millions of women worldwide. It would also be a crucial tool in understanding the progression of the disease, which can inform treatment decisions. Furthermore, it has implications for women's fertility, as endometriosis is a leading cause of infertility. Knowing whether and to what extent a woman has endometriosis can guide fertility treatments and increase the chances of successful pregnancy.

In essence, Hera Biotech's mission and our diagnostic test are about empowering women with knowledge about their own bodies, giving them more control over their health and treatment options, and ultimately improving their overall well-being. It's about time that researchers dedicate time and funding to understanding the basic biology of endometriosis.

## Christine Metz, PhD, Professor at Feinstein Institutes for Medical Research Northwell Health ROSE Study

*The Research OutSmarts Endometriosis (ROSE) study is an innovative approach to researching endometriosis, aiming to identify genetic markers of the disease. Episode 203 aired April 5, 2023.*

### What is the ROSE study?

The ROSE study, which stands for Research OutSmarts Endometriosis, was cofounded in 2013 by myself and my collaborator, Dr. Peter Gregersen, a geneticist at the Feinstein Institutes at Northwell Health. Our primary mission is to advance our understanding of endometriosis, aiming to develop more effective treatments and diagnostics for those affected by this condition. To address the significant issues of the current lack of well-tolerated treatments and the extensive delay in diagnosis—which averages seven to ten years primarily due to the need for surgical intervention for a definitive diagnosis—we've taken a novel approach by focusing on the study of menstrual effluent, or menstrual blood.

This decision was based on the understanding that the endometrial-like tissues growing outside of the uterus in individuals with endometriosis could provide invaluable insights when studied through menstrual blood. We observed that the cells lining the uterus of those with endometriosis differ significantly from those in healthy controls, showcasing more inflammatory cell types and fewer uterine natural killer cells. These findings suggest a distinct inflammatory profile in individuals with endometriosis, which could be pivotal in developing noninvasive diagnostic methods and novel treatments.

Our approach involves participants collecting their menstrual blood using a menstrual cup or a novel external sponge we developed, which is then shipped to our laboratory for analysis. This process allows us to study menstrual blood in the privacy and comfort of the participant's home. Despite some skepticism, our work has garnered significant interest and participation, with over 5,000 menstruators enrolled to date, showcasing the community's eagerness to contribute to this important research.

### What is menstrual effluent and why could it be useful for diagnosing uterine diseases?

Menstrual effluent is essentially menstrual blood, though it's not quite identical to peripheral blood—it has a slightly different composition. Scientifically, we use this term to represent the complex mixture of cells, tissues, and secretions expelled during menstruation. Surprisingly, before our work with the ROSE study, no one, to our knowledge, had extensively studied menstrual blood for any uterine health conditions or women's health in general, despite its direct relevance.

This oversight seems bewildering. Menstrual blood has the potential to provide insights into a variety of uterine conditions, including endometriosis. The lack of prior studies on menstrual effluent could be attributed to the societal and medical stigma surrounding menstruation. Even within the medical community, engaging directly with menstrual blood is something that causes hesitation. I have encountered physicians who are uncomfortable asking their patients to contribute menstrual blood for research. This stigma undermines the potential for significant scientific and medical advancements.

With continued research and the potential future approval by the FDA, we aim to make menstrual blood analysis a standard part of annual exams, offering a "treasured window" into uterine and reproductive health that has been overlooked for far too long. We may even be able to identify signals for other uterine health conditions such as fibroids.

## Sateria Venable, Founder and CEO at Fibroid Foundation

*Fibroid Foundation's mission is to amplify the voices of women living with fibroids. They intentionally create and support initiatives to find a cure for fibroids by advocating for ongoing research funding.*
*Episode 86 aired February 1, 2021.*

### What is a uterine fibroid?

Uterine fibroids are noncancerous, muscular tumors in the uterus, varying in size from a pea to as large as a watermelon. They are incredibly common, with up to 70 percent of women diagnosed by age fifty, and the prevalence rises to 80 percent among women of color. Symptoms can range widely due to fibroids' "chameleon" nature; they might include heavy menstrual bleeding, pain, fatigue from bleeding leading to anemia, and discomfort in various forms such as back or leg pain. Notably, fibroids can also be asymptomatic.

Diagnosis is typically achieved through ultrasound and pelvic exams, with MRI being the gold standard for determining a fibroid's precise location and blood supply before surgery. Treatment options vary, often starting with hormone-based medications like birth control pills to manage symptoms. However, these treatments don't halt disease progression and mainly target symptom relief. In severe cases, surgical options are presented, which historically, and alarmingly, have included total hysterectomy as a primary suggestion. This approach is now considered unacceptable without offering all available treatment options, aiming to preserve the uterus and fertility whenever possible.

**How could you get funding passed in the US government for fibroid research?**

Advocating for uterine fibroid research on Capitol Hill involved establishing common ground, especially when engaging with male staffers in their twenties. So, we used the National Defense Authorization Act to convey the importance of researching uterine fibroids. Thousands of women in the military suffer from uterine fibroids and require crucial support. By leveraging the argument that a significant portion of our armed forces need special care and cannot perform at their highest capacity due to fibroids, we hoped to convince enough folks in the capital to allocate additional funding to research fibroids.

The breakthrough came with the introduction of a fibroid bill, championed in the Senate by Senator Kamala Harris and in the House by Congresswoman Yvette Clarke. This significant milestone bill promises four years of funding for fibroid research at NIH, allocating $30 million annually.

Until we have more women in leadership positions and until these topics are destigmatized and men realize how common and interrupting these conditions are, we must find common ground to make win-win situations. This funding is going toward new innovations to detect and treat uterine fibroids at the source.

## Kim Rodriguez, Cofounder and Former CEO at Acessa Health

*Acessa Health created the Acessa ProVu system, a fully integrated laparoscopic system that combines radiofrequency ablation with advanced intra-abdominal ultrasound visualization and guidance mapping. This enables physicians to effectively and safely treat women with symptomatic, benign uterine fibroids. Episode 72 aired December 16, 2020.*

### How common are uterine fibroids, and what are the current treatments?

A uterine fibroid, a benign growth in the uterus, ranges from blueberry to a grapefruit in size, varying in number and location—inside the uterus, within the uterine muscle, or outside. Affecting 70-80 percent of women, with only a third experiencing symptoms, women of color are four times more likely to be affected than White women, making it significant. The current standard involves major surgery—a hysterectomy or myomectomy—both requiring a six- to eight-week recovery time and impacting the uterus.

Typical symptoms in a fibroid patient include heavy menstrual bleeding, abdominal pain, urinary pain, and painful sex—a debilitating condition often not discussed. Women with uterine fibroids can experience prolonged bleeding for ten to twenty years, along with pain. Some may appear pregnant or overweight due to fibroids causing these changes.

Over 60 percent of hysterectomies are unnecessary, and this fact presents an opportunity for change. The top surgical procedures for women are C-sections and hysterectomies—two potentially unnatural interventions.

In the southern states, there's a significantly higher rate of hysterectomies. For example, with its predominantly Hispanic population, women in San Antonio, Texas, have far more fibroids than in Austin. Conversely, women in Denver, Colorado, who are mostly White, report the fewest fibroids. The reasons still need to be fully understood, but it's an issue. Lower socioeconomic areas, especially in the South, face challenges in obtaining insurance coverage for new therapies and innovations. For our procedure, securing a category one CPT code required fighting payer by payer for approval. We successfully obtained coverage in Texas, Illinois, Maryland, DC, and other states, with major carriers like Aetna and Blue Cross Blue Shield. However, southern states like Louisiana, Alabama, and Tennessee remain holdouts, which is puzzling given their high rates of hysterectomies.

### How does the Acessa technology work?

Acessa is a technology that applies radiofrequency ablation or heat in a minimally invasive way to treat individual fibroids. It's a two-port laparoscopic procedure, performed on an outpatient basis under anesthesia. A percutaneous needle targets each fibroid, treating all of them without requiring cutting and suturing into the uterus. After the procedure, the patient typically goes home the same day and can return to normal activities in about three to five days.

Fibroids can be filled with blood, making them squishy or calcific and hard like baseballs. Acessa, in its treatment by applying heat to these individual fibroids, transforms the hard fibroid into a softer, marshmallow-like texture. Over time, the treated fibroid begins to shrink and gets absorbed within the tissue. As a result, both the uterus and the fibroid reduce in size.

* * *

In wrapping up our exploration into the vast and intricate landscape of uterine health, it's evident that the path to understanding and effectively managing conditions like endometriosis, adenomyosis, uterine fibroids, and uterine cancer is paved with innovation, perseverance, and collaboration. From Hera Biotech's groundbreaking nonsurgical diagnostic test that promises to revolutionize how endometriosis is identified and staged, to the ROSE study's novel approach of studying menstrual effluent to uncover the genetic markers of disease, the frontier of uterine health research is expanding. The Fibroid Foundation's tireless advocacy has placed fibroid research on the congressional radar and highlighted the power of patient voices in driving change. Meanwhile, Acessa Health's minimally invasive solution for fibroids points toward a future where treatment can be as personalized as the conditions it aims to conquer. These narratives underscore the urgency of addressing women's health issues and illuminate the potential for significant advancements when we dare to challenge the status quo. As we continue to navigate this complex terrain, let us draw inspiration from these pioneers, recognizing that the journey toward better uterine health is one we embark on together, armed with knowledge, compassion, and the unwavering belief in a healthier future for all women.

# Chapter 3
# Vaginal and Urinary Health

**AMY, A WOMAN IN HER LATE TWENTIES** with aspirations that soared high on the corporate ladder, found herself grappling with an unseen adversary that was as persistent as it was painful. Despite her best efforts to focus and excel in her career, recurring vaginal infections became a relentless distraction, each episode leaving her in excruciating discomfort as if her body was in a constant state of betrayal. The burning sensation made it almost impossible to maintain her composure during crucial meetings and presentations, casting a shadow over her professional demeanor. Every visit to the doctor ended with the same prescription: another round of antibiotics, which offered only temporary relief before the cycle of infection and discomfort resumed. Amy suspected the root of her troubles lay in the IUD she had chosen for its convenience, theorizing that a biofilm might have formed around it. Still, her concerns were dismissed by her doctors with a patronizing skepticism. How could a woman so focused on her business career possibly understand the complexities of medical biofilms?

Frustrated and increasingly desperate, Amy's journey through the medical system felt like a maze with no exit. Each dismissal from a doctor, each condescending rebuke, chipped away at her hope for a solution. It wasn't until a year had passed, after consulting with six different physicians, that she finally encountered a doctor who listened—took her symptoms and her suspicions seriously—and agreed to remove the IUD. With the removal of the IUD and a final course of antibiotics, Amy experienced a relief that felt almost foreign after so long. The infections ceased, allowing her to reclaim her health and focus again on her career aspirations without the constant, fiery distraction. This experience, while challenging, reinforced Amy's trust in her understanding of her body, underscoring the importance of perseverance and advocacy in one's health journey.

Urinary and vaginal health are critical aspects of a woman's overall well-being. Various conditions such as urinary tract infections (UTIs), yeast infections, bacterial vaginosis (BV), and sexually transmitted infections (STIs) significantly impact women's lives. Alarmingly, the misuse of hygiene products has further exacerbated these health issues, introducing harmful chemicals into women's bodies.

The vagina, which is like the eyeball in that it is self-cleaning, maintains health through a balance of good and bad bacteria. Disruptions in this balance, caused by factors like antibiotics, douching, or hormonal changes, can lead to various issues.[33] Vaginal discharge, often a sign of imbalance, varies in appearance and odor depending on health status. Unhealthy discharge is typically distinct in color and smell as increasing discharge volume is a technique of the vagina to push out impurities.[34]

Up to 75 percent of women will experience at least one yeast infection in their lifetime.[35] BV affects 29.2 percent of women aged fourteen to forty-nine in the US.[36] Over one million STIs are acquired every day worldwide, with chlamydia, gonorrhea, trichomoniasis, and syphilis accounting for most cases.[37]

These conditions can lead to discomfort, stress, and, in severe cases, complications in pregnancy and increased risk of acquiring other STIs, including HIV. The psychological impact and physical discomfort often lead to a reduced quality of life.

Proper diagnosis is crucial for effective treatment. For yeast infections, over-the-counter antifungal treatments are often sufficient. However, BV requires prescription antibiotics. Misdiagnosis is common, with about 62 percent of women mistaking BV for a yeast infection before proper diagnosis.[38]

UTIs, particularly common in women, are often caused by bacteria entering the urinary tract. More than 50 percent of women will experience at least one UTI in their lifetime.[39] Recurrent UTIs, defined as multiple infections within a year, require specific medical attention and possibly long-term antibiotic treatment.

Women are up to thirty times more likely than men to develop UTIs.[40] About four in ten women who experience a UTI will have another within six months.[41]

Factors such as sexual activity, certain birth control methods, pregnancy, menopause, and medical conditions like diabetes increase the risk. Common symptoms include pain during urination, frequent urges to urinate, and abdominal pressure. If untreated, UTIs can lead to kidney infections and other serious health issues.

Many feminine hygiene products contain hazardous chemicals like carcinogens, reproductive toxins, and allergens. This exposure is particularly concerning given the absorptive nature of vaginal tissue. Women of color and low socioeconomic status are disproportionately affected due to higher usage rates of certain products like douches and powders.[42]

Up to 86 percent of US women use tampons, exposing them to potentially harmful chemicals.[43] Black and Latina women are more likely to use products like douches, wipes, and sprays, increasing their risk of chemical exposure. Products like anti-itch creams often contain irritants or allergens, worsening symptoms.

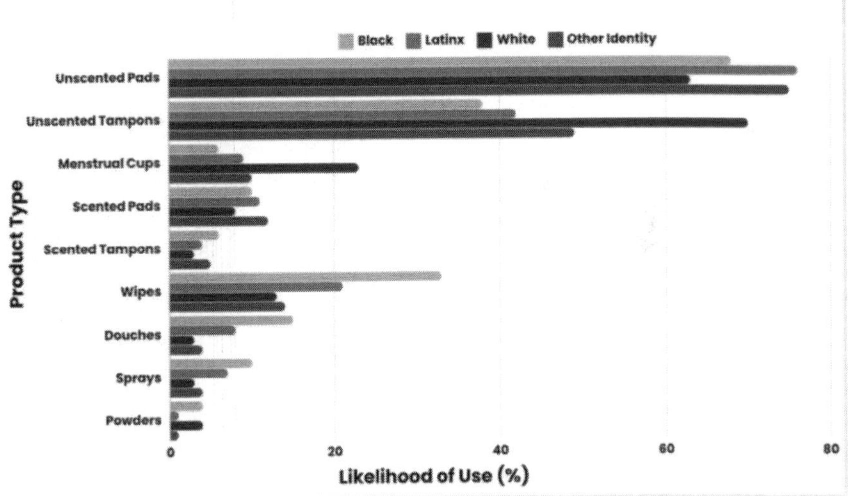


*Figure 8. Women of color are less likely to use unscented tampons and menstrual cups and more likely to use wipes and douches than White women.*[44]

Several companies are addressing these issues by creating products free of harmful chemicals and advocating for transparency in ingredient disclosure. These efforts aim to reduce the health risks associated with traditional feminine care products.

Urinary and vaginal health issues significantly impact women's lives, with various conditions affecting millions globally. Luckily innovators and researchers are taking vaginal and urinary health seriously and developing novel understanding and technologies to improve this vertical of women's health.

## Melissa Herbst-Kralovetz, PhD, Professor and Katherine Rhodes, PhD, Assistant Professor at University of Arizona

*Dr. Katherine Rhodes researches bacterial adaptation in sexually transmitted infections in the female reproductive tract. Dr. Melissa Herbst-Kralovetz studies the correlation between vaginal dysbiosis and the progression of gynecologic disease into cancer and other conditions. Episode 195 aired February 8, 2023.*

### What is the relationship between the vaginal microbiome and STIs?

The vaginal microbiome plays a crucial role in women's reproductive health, particularly in the context of STIs. It's a complex ecosystem primarily dominated by lactobacilli, which are beneficial bacteria that help maintain a healthy vaginal environment. These bacteria contribute to the acidity of the vagina, creating an environment that's generally hostile to pathogenic microbes.

However, when there's an imbalance or dysbiosis in the vaginal microbiome, it can lead to increased susceptibility to STIs. For instance, a decrease in lactobacilli and an overgrowth of other, less beneficial bacteria can create conditions that favor the transmission and colonization of pathogens like *Neisseria gonorrhoeae*, the bacteria responsible for gonorrhea, and others causing chlamydia or syphilis.

Additionally, conditions like BV, which is characterized by a dysbiotic vaginal microbiome, have been linked with a higher risk of acquiring STIs. BV alters the vaginal environment in a way that can compromise the natural defense mechanisms, making it easier for STIs to establish infection.

**What other health conditions could be influenced by the vaginal microbiome?**

The relationship between the vaginal microbiome and various health conditions, particularly cancer, is a fascinating and emerging area of research. For instance, in the case of cervical cancer, we know that the human papillomavirus (HPV) is a key causative agent. However, the presence of HPV alone is not sufficient to cause cancer. Research indicates that a dysbiotic vaginal microbiome may contribute to the persistence and progression of HPV infection toward cervical dysplasia and eventually cancer. Women with a healthy balance of lactobacilli are less likely to have persistent HPV infections and subsequent progression to cervical cancer.

Further research is exploring the connections between vaginal dysbiosis and other forms of gynecological cancers like endometrial cancer. The hypothesis is that certain pathogenic bacteria might ascend from the vagina to the upper reproductive tract, affecting the uterine lining and potentially contributing to carcinogenesis.

Now, regarding the relationship between the vaginal microbiome and the gut microbiome, this is a relatively new field of study but an intriguing one. The gut microbiome influences overall health, including mental health, immune function, and hormonal balance. There's a concept called the *estrobolome*, a collection of gut bacteria capable of metabolizing estrogens. These bacteria can significantly impact estrogen levels in the body, thus potentially influencing vaginal health and the vaginal microbiome.

Moreover, stress and lifestyle factors can impact both the gut and vaginal microbiomes. For instance, stress can lead to gut dysbiosis, which might indirectly affect the vaginal microbiome. These two microbiomes have a bidirectional relationship, mediated by systemic factors like immune responses and hormonal changes.

## Hana Janebdar, Founder and CEO at Juno Bio

*Juno Bio is developing an at-home vaginal microbiome sequencing test for women. This enables them to learn about their vaginal health and find adequate treatment plans with their healthcare provider for common conditions like yeast infection and BV. Episode 162 aired April 4, 2022.*

## Tell us about the vaginal microbiome.

A microbiome is a community of microbes that live and interact collectively, relying on each other within a specific environment. This perspective contrasts with focusing solely on individual microbes.

Discovering a significant gap in understanding and available products for women regarding the vaginal microbiome was surprising. Given its profound impact on billions of women, disruptions in the vaginal microbiome are often underestimated, and their implications run deep. Scientifically, the vaginal microbiome's mechanistic relationships with associated conditions are more substantial than those of the gut microbiome, presenting a compelling avenue for meaningful research and development.

Literature provides some insight into what a healthy vaginal microbiome looks like, acknowledging a strong ethnic component. The definition of *healthy* varies among ethnic groups, introducing nuances into characterizing a healthy state. The vaginal microbiome affects the way women live, which can be influenced by factors such as ethnicity, menopause, and menstrual cycles. While there's relative stability compared to the gut microbiome, ongoing characterization and learning are essential.

The origins of the vaginal microbiome remain a topic of exploration, with some indications that individuals are born with it or acquire it during specific life stages.

Lactobacillus, particularly *Lactobacillus crispatus* for Caucasian women and *Lactobacillus iners* for other ethnicities, plays a crucial role in maintaining a healthy vaginal microbiome. Lactobacilli produce lactic acid, creating an environment that hinders the survival of invading pathogens. Unlike the gut microbiome, where diversity is sought, the vagina benefits from a robust population of lactobacilli.

Disruption of the vaginal microbiome, often triggered by factors like antibiotic overuse or unprotected, penetrative sex, can lead to issues such as yeast infections, bacterial vaginosis, and urinary tract infections. Recurrent disruptions may stem from misdiagnosis or inadequate treatment. Conditions like BV affect a significant percentage of women annually, emphasizing the urgency of accurate diagnosis and effective treatment.

Ensuring proper diagnosis and treatment is crucial in preventing chronic or recurrent disruptions in the vaginal microbiome, highlighting the importance of addressing these issues accurately to enhance women's well-being.

### What does Juno Bio do?

Juno Bio is revolutionizing women's health through an at-home vaginal microbiome test, offering a comprehensive and personalized insight into the microbial composition of the vagina. The process involves receiving a kit, similar to a COVID test, swabbing the vagina for twenty seconds, and sending it back for analysis. Results are delivered within five to ten days. Following the results, individuals have the opportunity for a one-on-one session with a vaginal coach who addresses any questions. The anonymized data is also utilized for further research to bridge gender health gaps.

The current gold standard for vaginal microbiome testing is a culture-based test with fourteen criteria. However, this method has limitations as most bacteria cannot be cultured in the lab, providing an incomplete view of the microbial landscape. PCR (polymerase chain reaction) tests, while more advanced than the gold standard, have their challenges, especially in cases where conditions are not accurately characterized. This can result in negative test outcomes, incorrect diagnoses, and subsequently, high recurrence rates. Juno Bio utilizes next-generation sequencing, a superior approach, allowing the examination of all genetic material from the microbial sample, providing a more thorough and accurate understanding of the vaginal microbiome.

## Melissa Kramer, Founder and CEO at Live UTI Free

*Live UTI Free is a patient-advocacy and research organization with a highly engaged community. Episode 166 aired May 1, 2022.*

### What is a UTI and what puts women at risk of developing one?

A urinary tract infection, or UTI, is an infection occurring in any part of the urinary tract, including the urethra, bladder, ureters, and kidneys. Acute UTIs are severe with sudden onset, typically treated with antibiotics. However, the situation is more complicated when it comes to recurrent and chronic UTIs.

Chronic UTIs have a profound impact on a woman's life, affecting not just physical health but also mental well-being, relationships, and daily functioning. The recurring nature of the infection, coupled with a lack of effective long-term treatments, leads to significant frustration and emotional distress.

Statistics show that one in two women will experience a UTI in their lifetime, with a considerable percentage developing recurrent infections. The challenges in accurately diagnosing and effectively treating UTIs highlight the need for better medical understanding and more research in this field.

There are several key risk factors that can increase the likelihood of women developing a UTI. One of the primary factors is female anatomy. The female urethra is shorter and closer to the anus compared to males, which makes it easier for bacteria to enter the urinary tract. This anatomical difference is a significant contributor to why women are more prone to UTIs than men.

Another risk factor is sexual activity. Sexual intercourse can introduce bacteria into the urinary tract, increasing the chance of an infection. This is often referred to as "honeymoon cystitis" in some cases. Women need to urinate after sexual activity to help flush out any bacteria that may have been introduced.

Hormonal changes, particularly during menopause, also play a role. The decrease in estrogen levels can lead to changes in the urinary tract, making it more susceptible to infection. Similarly, during pregnancy, physiological changes can increase the risk of UTIs.

Additionally, certain types of birth control, especially those involving diaphragms or spermicidal agents, can increase UTI risk. They may contribute to bacterial growth or alter the natural bacterial flora of the vagina and urethra.

Personal hygiene practices can also be a factor. Wiping from back to front after using the toilet can spread bacteria from the anal area to the urethra. It's recommended to wipe from front to back to reduce this risk.

Other factors include a history of UTIs, certain medical conditions like diabetes, which can impair the immune system, and lifestyle elements such as poor hydration and diet.

## What is the standard of care for UTIs?

The standard of care for testing UTIs primarily involves urine culture, a test where a urine sample is sent to a lab to identify bacteria. However, this method is significantly flawed. The test was not designed for the complexity of diagnosing UTIs and often fails to detect a wide range of bacteria in the urinary tract. This inadequacy leads to misdiagnoses and inappropriate or ineffective treatments.

There is an urgent need for a comprehensive update of guidelines and medical education. Current medical training and guidelines fail to address the complexity and nuances of UTIs, especially chronic and recurrent ones. Medical school curricula often lack in-depth UTI education, and clinicians are not adequately equipped to manage these infections effectively. This gap in knowledge and understanding has serious implications for patient care and treatment outcomes.

Antibiotic resistance is a critical and growing concern in treating recurring UTIs. The frequent use of antibiotics for these infections has led to an increase in antibiotic-resistant bacteria. This resistance complicates treatment strategies, as standard antibiotics may no longer be effective against certain strains of bacteria causing the UTI. As a result, patients may experience persistent or worsening symptoms despite undergoing conventional antibiotic treatment.

The situation is compounded by the limited range of antibiotics available for UTIs. When bacteria become resistant to commonly prescribed drugs, clinicians face the challenge of finding alternative treatments, which are often limited and may have more side effects. This scenario not only puts the patient at risk of prolonged suffering but also increases the likelihood of the infection progressing to more serious conditions, such as kidney infections.

Moreover, the cycle of repeated antibiotic use and the development of resistant bacteria create a public health concern. It highlights the urgent need for new approaches in UTI treatment, including developing antibiotics targeting specific bacteria and alternative therapies that reduce reliance on antibiotics. What women need are more solutions that prevent UTIs from occurring in the first place.

## Jenna Ryan, Founder and CEO at Uqora

*Uqora addresses UTIs from end to end, from symptom relief products through to proactive care supplements. Uqora has helped hundreds of thousands of people get on top of their urinary health and is now available in retail stores across the USA. Episode 51 aired October 5, 2020.*

### What is Uqora, and why did you start it?

I started Uqora because I was a chronic UTI sufferer, and I was frustrated with the heavy rotation of antibiotics that seemed more like a bandage than a solution. With my partner, Spencer Gordon, a biochemist, we saw a need for research-backed, effective solutions for urinary tract health. A proactive approach was essential since UTIs affect half of all women and are the second most common infection. Since launching Uqora in 2017, we've helped over 50,000 women manage their UTIs.

Uqora offers a range of products focusing on urinary tract health, including symptom control for active infections, cleansing wipes, and our proactive care line, which includes a drink mix and two daily products. The drink mix is designed to flush the urinary tract after activities like sex or exercise, which can introduce bacteria. The other two products are a daily supplement to cleanse the bladder of biofilm and a vaginal probiotic to regulate urinary tract health. Our products are formulated based on the best clinical research available, offering women a scientifically sound alternative to managing their urinary tract health.

### Are peeing after sex and drinking cranberry juice effective ways to avoid UTIs?

Women are advised to pee after sex because it's an effective way to flush out bacteria that may have entered the urinary tract during intercourse. This action helps reduce the risk of developing a UTI, given our anatomical structure, particularly the short distance from the urethra to the bladder.

Cranberry juice's effectiveness in treating UTIs is a widely held belief, but research is inconclusive. While some studies suggest cranberry juice might have benefits, it's generally less effective than once thought. The American Medical Association published a study in 2016 debunking the cranberry myth for UTI treatment. Cranberry juice may be better than doing nothing, and it can help with hydration, but it's not a reliable solution for treating or preventing UTIs. There are a growing number of products like Uqora that are helping women prevent these UTIs such as vaginal-safe lubricants.

## Wendy Strgar, Founder and CEO at Good Clean Love

*Good Clean Love is a leading sexual wellness brand that produces natural products, including lubricants, aphrodisiacs, and other intimacy-enhancing items. Episode 225 aired January 3, 2024.*

## How do chemicals found in today's hygiene products affect a woman's vaginal health?

Many products in the market, unfortunately, contain harmful petrochemicals like propylene glycol and polyethylene glycol. These chemicals can significantly disrupt the delicate balance of the vaginal microbiome, leading to issues like bacterial vaginosis and other vaginal health problems.

Hyperosmolar lubricants can pull moisture from vaginal cells, causing the protective top layer to slough off within four hours. This increases susceptibility to bacterial vaginosis by 60 percent as the healthy lactobacilli cannot maintain a pH balance. Long-term dysbiosis from chemical-heavy products can lead to conditions like vulvodynia and inflammation. Treating resulting infections with antibiotics only creates more issues by killing beneficial bacteria without restoring the healthy biome.

Understanding the impact of these chemicals is crucial. They create an environment prone to dysbiosis, making the vagina more susceptible to infections and diseases. It's important to advocate for the use of natural, organic alternatives. Products designed to mimic the body's natural secretions are key to supporting and maintaining a healthy vaginal microbiome.

Educating and empowering women to understand the ingredients in their hygiene products is essential for making informed choices. As someone deeply invested in the field of women's health and sexual wellness, I am committed to creating products that are not only effective but also safe for women's bodies. It's about prioritizing vaginal health and offering solutions that align with the body's natural functions and needs.

## What is Good Clean Love and why did you start it?

Good Clean Love began as a personal quest to address my own intimate health issues. Frustrated with the petrochemical-based products prescribed by doctors, which caused severe reactions, I embarked on a mission to create natural, body-friendly products. My experience resonated with countless other women facing similar challenges, highlighting a significant gap in the market for safe, effective intimate care products.

The uniqueness of Good Clean Love lies in its formulation. Unlike many conventional products laden with harmful chemicals, Good Clean Love products are designed with the health of the vaginal microbiome in mind. Like the flagship, organic lubricants, our products are free from harsh petrochemicals and feature natural ingredients like aloe vera. This approach not only reduces the risk of irritation and adverse reactions but also supports the delicate balance of the vaginal ecosystem.

## Mitchella Gilbert, MBA, CEO at Oya Femtech Apparel

*Oya has revolutionized performance wear to prevent recurrent vulva, vaginal, and urinary tract infections caused by exercise.*
*Episode 89 aired February 10, 2021.*

### Tell us about how leggings and yoga pants today are affecting vaginal health?

Current leggings and yoga pants, while popular for their comfort and style, unfortunately have a downside when it comes to vaginal health. The primary issue is the material used—typically spandex or similar synthetic fabrics. These materials are known for trapping moisture and heat close to the body, creating an environment that fosters bacterial growth.

When you wear tight-fitting leggings or yoga pants, especially for extended periods or during intense physical activities, they can restrict airflow to the vaginal area. This lack of ventilation leads to increased sweat and moisture being held against the skin, which can disrupt the natural balance of bacteria in the vaginal area. This moist, warm environment often exacerbates yeast infections and bacterial vaginosis.

Moreover, many women, especially athletes or those leading active lifestyles, spend significant time in these leggings. This prolonged exposure only increases the risk of developing such vaginal health issues. It's not just about the discomfort but also about the potential long-term implications for one's health.

At Oya, we recognize this problem and are addressing it by rethinking the design and materials of our leggings. Our goal is to offer women a healthier alternative that allows for better breathability and moisture control without sacrificing comfort or style. We believe it's crucial to balance all these aspects to promote overall well-being and health in women's activewear.

### What are Oya leggings?

Oya leggings is a revolutionary approach to women's activewear, especially focusing on health and comfort. Born at UCLA and developed in a fashion lab, we at Oya are obsessed with engineering apparel that looks good and promotes feminine health. Our leggings are designed to be breathable, leak-absorbent, and offer contour shaping. The idea behind Oya leggings is to support women throughout their day comfortably, providing them with an apparel choice sensitive to their health needs.

We understand that traditional sportswear often overlooks the unique requirements of a woman's body. Standard leggings, for instance, can increase the likelihood of vaginal health issues due to moisture-trapping materials like spandex. Oya leggings are different. We have reimagined the design to include features like breathable fabric and a removable cotton pad that absorbs moisture, keeping the vaginal area dry and healthy.

Our leggings are not just a piece of clothing; they represent a shift in how women's activewear is perceived and designed. It's not just about looking good but feeling good and staying healthy. Oya leggings are a testament that comfort, style, and health can coexist in women's fashion. We are committed to creating a community around the idea of supporting feminine health with functional apparel.

* * *

Here we have uncovered the intricacies of women's health issues that, while commonly experienced, often need to be discussed and addressed. This chapter illuminates the critical importance of understanding and maintaining the delicate balance of the vaginal microbiome, the alarming prevalence of UTIs, and the detrimental effects of certain hygiene products on vaginal and urinary health. These conversations highlight the significance of accurate diagnosis, the challenges of antibiotic resistance, and the importance of avoiding harmful chemicals in feminine hygiene products. Moreover, developing new technologies and natural product alternatives showcases a promising shift toward safer, more effective treatments and preventive measures tailored to women's unique health needs. We are advocating for a future where these crucial aspects of women's well-being are no longer sidelined but are recognized as integral to their overall health and quality of life.

# Chapter 4
# Sexual Health

**NAOMI FOUND HERSELF AT THE HEART** of an ever-widening chasm within her marriage, a chasm deepened by her struggle with diminished sexual desire. This struggle wasn't just a private battle; it had become the focal point of contention between her and her husband, who attributed their deteriorating relationship to her apparent lack of interest in sex. She remembered a time when arousal wasn't such a foreign concept and when intimacy with her husband was something she actively craved rather than avoided. Now, however, the thought of sex left her feeling drained, devoid of any desire or energy. Their disconnection grew more palpable each month, a silent testament to their fading closeness. The weight of blame settled heavily on her shoulders, both from her husband's accusations and her own self-criticism. Naomi couldn't shake off the feeling that something was fundamentally wrong with her, that perhaps she was failing as a partner and a woman.

Compounding her distress was a secret she harbored close to her chest—a secret she had never shared with her husband. Despite their years of intimacy, Naomi had never experienced an orgasm. Each encounter had ended with her feigning satisfaction, a performance aimed at bolstering her husband's ego, sparing his feelings, and an act of desperation to do sex "correctly." She clung to the hope that maybe, just maybe, if she pretended well enough, her body would eventually learn to find pleasure. Yet, as time passed, this hope faded into resignation. The realization that she wasn't even sure what an orgasm should feel like left her feeling even more isolated and defective. This internal turmoil was exacerbated by the pervasive narrative in media that normalized her experience, suggesting that disinterest in sex was an inherent part of long-term relationships for women. Naomi found herself wondering if this disconnect, this absence of pleasure, was simply what marriage entailed, or if perhaps, beyond the veil of societal expectations and conjugal obligations, there might be a path to rediscovering intimacy and desire on her own terms.

Historically, women's sexual health has been enshrouded in taboo across various cultures worldwide, leading to a profound misunderstanding and underrepresentation in the broader narrative of female existence. This social stigma, deeply rooted in patriarchal norms, has perpetuated a cycle where women's sexual desires have been vilified, and their pleasure largely dismissed or ignored, fostering a culture where men's sexuality has been central. The late 1960s marked a pivotal era as the feminist movement gained momentum, challenging not only their exclusion from politics and the workforce but also the traditional sexual roles imposed on women. The sexual revolution, fueled by feminists' push for recognition of women's sexual needs and rights to pleasure, sparked intense debates between feminists advocating for empowerment and social conservatives who viewed these changes as a threat to societal structures.

Despite the strides made since Marie Stopes's 1918 groundbreaking book, *Married Love*, which included advice on maintaining a satisfying and pleasurable sex life in a marriage, modern society continues to grapple with many of the same issues regarding women's sexual health and agency. The persistence of slut-shaming, victim-blaming in sexual assault cases, and ongoing battles over reproductive rights underscore the enduring challenges. Additionally, the prevailing orgasm gap, the rising interest in cosmetic genital surgeries, and the multifaceted levels of discrimination faced by women from diverse backgrounds, genders, and sexual orientations highlight the complexities of addressing women's sexual health in today's world. Although significant progress has been made toward acknowledging and fulfilling women's sexual rights, the journey toward fully dismantling centuries-old stigmas and achieving true understanding and equality in sexual health remains ongoing. It is imperative to confront and address the shame and silence surrounding women's sexuality, empowering all women to speak openly about their health, preferences, and needs without fear of judgment or retribution.

SexTech, at its core, is an innovative intersection of technology and human sexuality. It's a dynamic field that encompasses a range of technologies aimed at enhancing, innovating, and revolutionizing the sexual experience. This goes beyond just physical pleasure; it touches on aspects of health, well-being, education, safety, gender identity, and even social interactions related to sexuality.

SexTech includes a vast array of technologies ranging from software applications that provide sexual education or improve intimate connections, to hardware like advanced sex toys and medical devices aimed at sexual health and wellness. It also includes cutting-edge technologies like virtual reality (VR) and artificial intelligence (AI), which open new possibilities for sexual experiences and connections. AI can tailor sexual wellness programs or suggest products based on individual preferences and needs. VR, on the other hand, is creating virtual environments for the safe exploration of fantasies, enhancing long-distance relationships, or even providing therapeutic sexual experiences.

In the medical world, SexTech is being used to treat sexual dysfunctions and enhance sexual health. This includes devices designed for physical therapy of sexual organs, products that aid in overcoming sexual health challenges, and even telemedicine platforms that offer confidential consultations with sexual health professionals.

An often-overlooked aspect of SexTech is its role in personal safety and consent in sexual encounters. Technologies are being developed to ensure safer dating experiences and to facilitate clear communication of consent, making sexual interactions not only more enjoyable but also safer for all parties involved.

SexTech is not just a collection of products and services, it's a movement that reflects and influences societal attitudes toward sexuality. By normalizing conversations about sexual health and pleasure, SexTech plays a crucial role in promoting a more open, inclusive, and healthy perspective on sexuality in society.

The "pleasure gap" refers to the disparity in sexual satisfaction and orgasm frequency between different genders and sexual orientations. It primarily highlights the gap between men and women, particularly in heterosexual encounters. Studies consistently show that while men reach orgasm in most of their sexual encounters, women experience this far less frequently.[45] This discrepancy is not just a matter of physical experience; it's deeply rooted in cultural, educational, and psychological factors.

Historically, male pleasure has often been prioritized in sexual encounters, with female pleasure being either ignored or misunderstood. Media portrayals, lack of comprehensive sex education, and enduring myths about female sexuality reinforce this imbalance.

Educational initiatives are crucial in closing the pleasure gap. Comprehensive sex education that goes beyond the basics of reproduction and focuses on pleasure, consent, and communication can empower individuals with the knowledge they need for fulfilling sexual experiences. This includes understanding the anatomy of pleasure, such as the clitoris's role in female orgasm.

The pleasure gap also has a psychological dimension. Women may feel less entitled to sexual pleasure or may not feel comfortable communicating their needs and desires. Encouraging open and honest communication between partners can lead to more satisfying sexual experiences. Understanding and addressing internalized beliefs about sexuality is essential for both partners to fully engage and enjoy their sexual experiences.

The landscape of research in female sexual wellness has been historically biased toward male-centric studies, leading to a substantial knowledge gap in understanding female sexuality. Fortunately, recent years have seen a surge in inclusive and detailed studies on female sexual health. This includes exploring the physiological, hormonal, and psychological factors affecting female arousal, desire, and satisfaction. For example, one study indicated that 43 percent of women reported symptoms of sexual dysfunction.[46]

The path to understanding female sexual wellness is riddled with challenges like societal stigmas, limited funding, and a lack of diverse participation in studies. This is compounded by the subjective nature of sexual wellness and the myriad of influencing factors, making standardized research difficult. The integration of technology in research has opened new avenues for collecting data. Online surveys and health apps are instrumental in gathering large-scale information, providing anonymity and convenience to participants. These digital platforms are critical in ensuring diversity and inclusivity in research demographics.

Research is increasingly focusing on disorders like hypoactive sexual desire disorder (HSDD), arousal disorders, and sexual pain disorders. A comprehensive approach, combining pharmacological treatments and nonpharmacological methods like psychotherapy, is being explored.

An emerging area of interest is the effect of chronic conditions and medications such as SSRIs (selective serotonin reuptake inhibitors) on female sexual health. Conditions like diabetes and cardiovascular diseases are linked to higher incidences of sexual dysfunction in women.

Future research is geared toward personalizing medical approaches to female sexual wellness. This includes understanding the long-term impacts of contraceptives, the influence of mental health, and the effectiveness of various treatments. Female sexual dysfunction (FSD) is a prevalent and multifaceted issue that affects a substantial portion of the female population. It encompasses a range of problems including disorders of desire, arousal, orgasm, and sexual pain, each contributing to personal distress and impacting quality of life, interpersonal relationships, and overall mental health.

The societal stigma and psychosocial factors heavily influence the reporting and understanding of FSD. Many women do not seek medical attention due to these barriers, further compounding the issue. This is reflected in the discrepancy between the high prevalence of reported symptoms and the lower rate of those seeking help.

Despite the high prevalence of FSD, research and treatment for male sexual dysfunction, such as erectile dysfunction, have historically received more attention. This discrepancy highlights a gender bias in both research and healthcare provisions, underscoring the need for more gender-specific research and treatment options.

In response to these disparities, SexTech companies are making incredible strides in improving female sexual wellness.

## Lyndsey Harper, MD, Founder and CEO at Rosy

*Rosy is a sexual wellness app created to address the gaps in resources for women experiencing low sexual desire. Episode 3 aired April 13, 2020.*

### What does Rosy offer women?

Rosy is a groundbreaking mobile platform dedicated to enhancing women's sexual wellness, especially those experiencing low sexual desire. As an ob-gyn, I was confronted with the lack of resources and support for women facing sexual wellness issues. This inspired me to create Rosy, a space where women can find evidence-based, accessible solutions.

Our app focuses on a holistic approach to sexual wellness, offering a range of tools designed to educate and empower women. The features include educational videos that provide insights into female sexuality, addressing common misconceptions and promoting a deeper understanding of women's sexual health. We emphasize the importance of knowing and respecting one's body, including correct anatomical knowledge and understanding the natural variations in sexual desire.

A unique aspect of Rosy is our curated library of erotica, developed with a focus on women's perspectives and experiences. Recognizing that mental stimulation plays a crucial role in sexual desire, our erotica collection is designed to cater to diverse preferences, allowing women to explore their sexuality in a safe, positive environment.

We've also introduced a community feature that enables women to connect, share experiences, and offer support to each other. This community aspect is crucial in breaking the silence and stigma surrounding women's sexual wellness.

Since its inception, Rosy has made significant strides, partnering with healthcare professionals and reaching thousands of women. Our mission is to bridge the gap in women's sexual healthcare, providing resources that are not only informative but also engaging and relevant to women's lives.

## Are there discrepancies between resources for male and female sexual wellness?

In the realm of sexual wellness, there's a striking disparity between the resources available for men and women, which is evident in healthcare, media representation, and funding.

Starting with healthcare, men have clearly defined pathways for addressing sexual dysfunction. Urologists are the go-to specialists for male sexual issues, and there's a well-established understanding and treatment protocol for conditions like erectile dysfunction. In contrast, female sexual wellness, particularly issues like low sexual desire, is often overlooked or inadequately addressed in medical training. This leaves a significant gap in healthcare for women, as many ob-gyns and general practitioners aren't equipped with the necessary tools or knowledge to effectively treat these concerns.

In the media, the discrepancy is also glaring. Erectile dysfunction and male sexual health are openly discussed and marketed, with a plethora of advertisements and educational materials. However, female sexual wellness is frequently shrouded in stigma and misinformation. Attempts to promote female sexual wellness or empowerment often face censorship or backlash, suggesting a societal discomfort with acknowledging and supporting women's sexual health.

Funding disparities further exacerbate these issues. Male-focused sexual health companies and products tend to receive more attention and investment from the pharmaceutical industry and venture capitalists. This is in stark contrast to the female sexual wellness sector, which struggles to attract similar levels of interest and investment. This funding gap not only hampers innovation in female sexual wellness but also reflects a broader societal trend of undervaluing women's health issues.

The challenge we face in bridging these discrepancies is not just about creating equitable resources but also about changing societal perceptions and attitudes toward female sexuality. It's about recognizing that women's sexual wellness is a vital aspect of their overall health and deserves the same attention, research, and investment as men's sexual health.

## Bryony Cole, Founder at Future of SexTech

*Bryony Cole hosts* The Future of Sex *Podcast, where she explores the innovative realm of SexTech and is the founder of SexTech School, the first sexual wellness accelerator. Episode 147 aired December 29, 2021.*

### How has SexTech evolved?

SexTech's existence mirrors human innovation throughout history, serving as a tool to address various needs. The emphasis doesn't need to revolve around high-tech solutions like AI or VR, especially within sexual wellness, where ancient artifacts like stone dildos from 35,000 years ago highlight the enduring nature of this industry.

Significant shifts have occurred due to evolving societal attitudes. Increased openness about sexuality, even during a pandemic, has heightened awareness of intimacy and its connection to overall health. The isolation experienced in recent times has underscored the importance of discussing sexuality and intimacy leading to a silver lining in these challenging times. This change in societal perception has affected media and everyday conversations and impacted investments in SexTech products.

Regarding product innovation, particularly in areas like robotics and adult entertainment, the #MeToo and Time's Up movements have brought more women into the industry. This shift has prompted changes in marketing strategies, moving away from traditional provocative imagery to educational approaches. Brands like Dame, Unbound, Rosewell, and even Goop have incorporated sex education into their messaging, making it more acceptable and less stigmatized.

Moreover, high-end and department stores now stock SexTech products, often alongside beauty items. This marketing strategy has changed the placement and accessibility of products like vulva creams, dildos, and lubricants. However, it's important to note that such changes can also come with issues of privilege and affordability.

A significant highlight in this evolving landscape is the focus on communication, storytelling, and the movement around female pleasure. Many individuals, regardless of technical expertise, are driven to the SexTech industry by personal experiences, breaking the isolation and loneliness often associated with sexual issues.

For the future of SexTech, the key lies in changing societal views on sexuality, reducing judgment and shame, and fostering openness. Increased investment in the industry will enable the creation of products and services catering to diverse niche audiences. Education, especially in the realm of sex education, plays a crucial role in breaking down barriers and addressing various sexual issues. The dream is to see innovation in sex education, potentially delivered through technology like robots or virtual reality, creating a safe and intimate learning environment. This focus on sex education is seen as a solution that can positively impact many aspects of sexual health and relationships, ultimately shaping a more open and informed future of SexTech. Such research will also help reshape perceptions of sex and how individuals experience and relate to sex.

## Cindy Gallop, Founder and CEO at Make Love Not Porn

*Make Love Not Porn is a social SexTech video-sharing platform that aims to facilitate healthy conversations about sex.*
*Episode 83 aired January 20, 2021.*

## What is MakeLoveNotPorn, and why did you start it?

I realized I was experiencing a convergence of two factors: easy access to explicit online content intersected with society's reluctance to openly discuss sex. When these two aspects aligned, it inadvertently turned porn into a form of sex education, but not in a positive way. I noticed various sexual behaviors in bed and understood their origin. If I was experiencing this, I thought others must be too. Remember, twelve or thirteen years ago, no one was addressing this issue. No one was writing about it. I felt compelled to take action. Eleven years ago, I created a rudimentary website, MakeLoveNotPorn.com, with minimal funding. Initially, it comprised only text, focusing on the contrast between the world of pornography and real-life experiences. I launched it in 2009, becoming the first TED speaker to utter explicit words on the TED stage. The talk went viral, generating an unexpected global response to my small website. I realized I had uncovered a significant global social problem. I received messages from a thousand individuals worldwide, sharing their experiences, regardless of age, gender, or sexual orientation. I felt a responsibility to expand MakeLoveNotPorn in a way that could make it more far-reaching, helpful, and effective. I transformed it into a business, MakeLoveNotPorn.tv, with a singular mission: making it easier for everyone worldwide to have open and honest conversations about sex. Our tagline is "pro-sex, pro-porn, pro-knowing the difference." We are the world's first user-generated, human-curated social platform for sharing sexual content. We resemble what Facebook would be if it allowed sexual self-expression. Our goal is to socialize and normalize sex in the real world, facilitating discussions, and promoting consent, communication, and positive sexual values and behavior. We aim to normalize and socialize real-world sex to facilitate discussions and promote consent, communication, healthy sexual values, and behaviors. We are at the forefront of what we call "the social sex revolution."

Sexuality is fluid, and MakeLoveNotPorn reflects this diversity in the real world. We break down barriers, embracing LGBTQIA+ inclusivity. Many of our contributors, whom we call MakeLoveNotPorn stars, had never recorded themselves engaging in sexual activities before joining us. They believe in our mission. Sharing their most intimate moments on our platform, even with strangers, often enhances their self-esteem and sexual self-perception. We provide education and practical demonstrations, including our popular lick-job videos, which are quick and effective tutorials on female pleasure. We are a communication medium, facilitating conversations about sex. Couples watch our videos together as a springboard for open and relaxed discussions.

As the only platform for sharing real-world sex videos, we offer numerous benefits. While porn resembles a Hollywood blockbuster, we are the documentary, providing a unique glimpse into how people have sex in the real world. This is valuable because social platforms are incredibly reassuring. We embrace real-world everything, from diverse body types to embracing accidents, awkwardness, and messiness. Watching real people enjoy themselves in bed, regardless of their body type, boosts body positivity and self-love. We believe that everybody is beautiful when having real-world sex, and it shows.

**What are the biggest challenges of SexTech companies?**

I tell everyone that we all have three fundamental boundaries: funding, access to infrastructure, and advertising ability. Solving the first one also addresses the other two, as the only way these obstacles disappear is when you provide substantial financial support. Raise enough funding to secure a significant advertising budget, and you'll be surprised at how rapidly these barriers vanish. Unfortunately, there are very few other viable solutions. As a founding member of SexTech, we've engaged in various efforts, such as lobbying and protesting outside Facebook's offices, and other ventures are making commendable strides with petitions. However, none of these actions will have a substantial impact. Money speaks volumes. When each of us possesses substantial advertising budgets, individually and collectively, these barriers will crumble.

We have only scratched the surface of what this category can become when we incorporate a female and diverse perspective. Currently, regrettably, when you mention "SexTech," people immediately think of sex toys and sex robots. They have yet to grasp this category's immense potential, including safe spaces to learn about sexuality.

## Andrea Barrica, Founder at O School

*O School is building a shame-free space by offering pleasure education through live streaming and moderated chat.*
*Episode 138 aired October 18, 2021.*

## What is O School, and why did you start it?

O School is an online platform that provides accessible, judgment-free, and science-based sexual education. I started it because there's a significant lack of comprehensive sexual education globally, and I wanted to create a safe space where people can learn about sexual wellness, pleasure, and intimacy.

O School began as a live-streaming platform for sexual education classes but evolved over time. We discovered that our audience needed more foundational education before attending classes. This realization guided us to focus on creating content that ranks well in search engines for specific, pleasure-related queries.

The unique aspect of O School is our approach to sex education. We address topics that are often overlooked by traditional medical resources but aren't explicitly pornographic. This balance allows us to serve a broad audience, including those seeking answers about pleasure, gender exploration, and intimacy.

## Why is customer acquisition such a large challenge for SexTech companies?

The customer acquisition challenges faced by SexTech companies are multifaceted and stem from various factors, including societal stigma, restrictive advertising policies, and the complexity of the market itself.

First, societal stigma around sexuality and sexual wellness creates a significant hurdle. This stigma leads to a general hesitancy in openly discussing or exploring these topics, which directly impacts how customers engage with SexTech products and services. The reluctance to openly discuss sexual wellness means that word of mouth, a powerful marketing tool for many industries, is less effective in the SexTech space.

Moreover, the advertising policies of major platforms like Facebook and Google need to be revised. These platforms often have strict guidelines about what constitutes acceptable content, severely limiting the ability of SexTech companies to advertise their products effectively. Even when allowed, the cost of advertising on these platforms can be prohibitively high due to the competition for ad space, leading to lower returns on investment.

The complexity of the market itself is another challenge. The SexTech industry is diverse, catering to various needs and preferences. This diversity means that companies must invest heavily in educating potential customers about their products and the broader context of sexual wellness. However, the ROI (return on investment) on educational content can be challenging to measure and often does not directly translate into sales.

Additionally, the SexTech market is still in its nascent stages, and channels for discovery and purchase need to be established. Unlike more mainstream products, SexTech items aren't typically sold in regular retail environments, which means companies have to work harder to find and engage their target audience.

Last, sustaining customer interest and retention is challenging. Many SexTech products, like vibrators, don't necessarily lend themselves to repeat purchases in short intervals, making it crucial for companies to diversify their product offerings or find ways to engage customers beyond the initial sale.

## Ti Chang, Cofounder and Chief Design Officer at Crave

*Crave is a lifestyle brand that designs discreet and luxurious sex toy vibrators. The company's first product was the Crave Duet, which was the first-ever crowdfunded sex toy. Episode 121 aired June 21, 2021.*

### Why did you want to design SexTech products?

I was drawn to addressing a very real human need—pleasure. The existing products meant to fulfill this need were poorly conceived, badly manufactured, and not designed with the users in mind. This raised two problems: product quality and the cultural stigma around these products. I aimed to create aesthetically pleasing and well-designed products that elevate the category and change the perception from gross to beautiful and empowering.

As a brand, we launched the world's first crowdfunded vibrator in 2011, followed by MyVibes in 2015, allowing users to customize vibration patterns. The feedback from users informed the final product. Our latest product, Duet Pro, takes customization to the next level. Pleasure is complicated, and our goal is to create products for various experiences, recognizing that there's no one-size-fits-all solution. We embrace diversity in pleasure, offering products suitable for different settings and experiences.

Our Vesper vibrator necklace, launched in 2014, stands out as a unique and patented product. It is an external vibrator for personal use and a stylish necklace for public wear. The Vesper has become a signature product for Crave, sparking conversations wherever it goes. Women share stories of wearing it to brunch or on their first Tinder dates, using it as a litmus test to gauge compatibility. The Vesper, with its elegant design, has contributed to Crave's recognition and success.

## Liz Klinger, Cofounder at Lioness

*Developer of a biometric, sensor-based vibrator paired with an application designed to guide women to understand, discover, and take control of their own bodies. Episode 42 aired September 2, 2020.*

### What is the history and current state of researching female sexual pleasure?

Historically, the conversation around sex, especially female pleasure, was almost nonexistent, either shrouded in taboo or skewed to focus predominantly on male pleasure. There was a huge component of human experience being ignored or misunderstood.

Pioneers like Masters and Johnson began exploring human sexuality in more scientific terms, but the specifics of female pleasure weren't the main focus. Much of the early research, even by them, was largely male-centric.

The challenges in this field are not just about societal taboos but institutional reluctance. Research in sexual health is tough due to bureaucracy and a bit of squeamishness from the academic and scientific communities. It's challenging to have sexual health discussions loudly in these circles.

Developing Lioness, a biofeedback vibrator, was groundbreaking in its approach to understanding sexual response. However, getting it recognized in certain scientific or health-related circles has been a journey. We were sometimes outright excluded from discussions in women's health-tech spaces because a product about sexual pleasure didn't fit the norm. This exclusion is both disappointing and ironic, given the integral role of sexual health in overall well-being.

Despite these challenges, the tide is slowly turning. There's growing recognition that understanding and exploring female sexual pleasure is essential for knowing the body, understanding health, and empowering individuals, which is why Lioness uses technology to enable the exploration and understanding of bodies better.

### How does Lioness contribute to female sexual research?

Lioness empowers individuals to explore and understand their own sexual responses through technology. We've developed a biofeedback vibrator that's not just about pleasure but also about gathering data on sexual response. This data is crucial because there's a significant gap in scientific knowledge about female sexual health and pleasure.

Our product uses advanced sensors to measure pelvic floor contractions, which are key indicators of sexual arousal and orgasm. This approach provides a unique and concrete way to visualize and understand orgasm patterns. By making this data accessible to users, we're demystifying aspects of female sexuality that have been poorly understood or ignored.

Furthermore, Lioness offers a platform for researchers to conduct studies on sexual health. By using the data collected from our devices, researchers can study various aspects of sexual health on a scale that's never been possible before. This is groundbreaking because small sample sizes and logistic challenges have limited traditional sexual health research. Lioness enables research on a much larger and diverse population, offering insights that can lead to more personalized understandings of sexual health and wellness.

## Soumyadip Rakshit, PhD, Cofounder and CEO at MysteryVibe

*MysteryVibe is the first brand whose vibrators are available to purchase with FSA and HSA cards due to their applications addressing health challenges such as pelvic pain and arousal disorder.*
*Episode 159 aired March 15, 2022.*

### How can vibrators improve physical health?

We use vibrators to address diverse sexual health issues. Our overarching goal is to unravel the positive impact of vibration therapy on sexual health, addressing specific conditions or concerns that affect both men and women.

We proved this hypothesis in our publication in the *Journal of Sexual Medicine* with our focus on topical genital-pelvic pain/penetration disorder (GPPPD). Through this study, we employed the Crescendo device three times a week, resulting in a remarkable five times improvement in pain scores over a three-month period. GPPPD, encompassing genital, pelvic, and penetration pain, holds significant importance in women's sexual health.

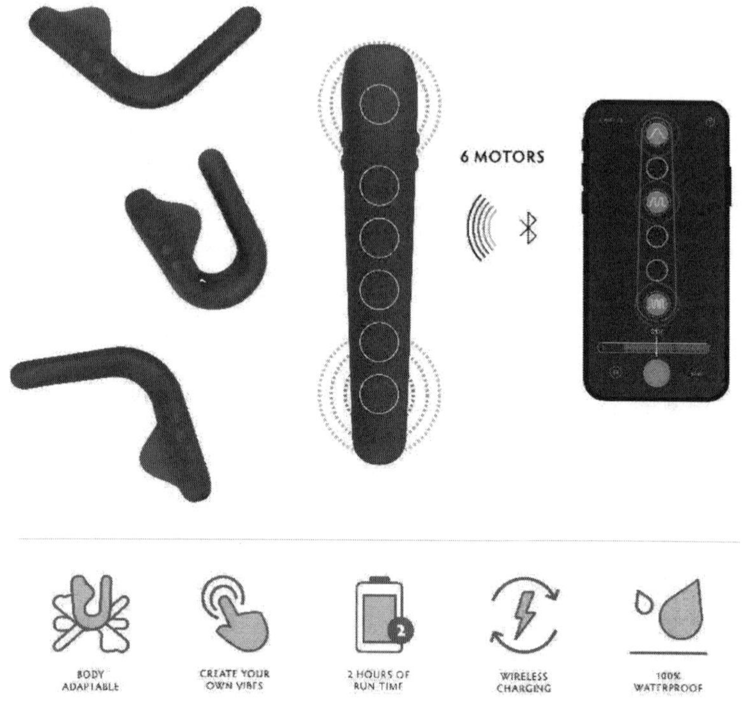


*Figure 9: MysteryVibe's Crescendo device significantly improved pelvic pain.*

Another study shifted the focus to period pain, employing an external vibrator application, such as placing it on the abdomen to deliver gentle vibrations. This approach aids in enhancing blood flow and alleviating pain. Our third study delves into arousal among perimenopausal and menopausal women, specifically before penetrative intercourse. The fourth study explores vestibulodynia, a form of vulvodynia, and investigates how varying vibration frequencies can alleviate pain associated with this condition.

## Is MysteryVibe a sexual wellness medical device or consumer product company?

In my experience, as a founder, navigating the decision-making process involves a crucial choice between strictly focusing on the medical aspects or embracing the broader spectrum of sexual wellness. The real challenge stems from the societal stigma and taboo surrounding pleasure, making fundraising and digital marketing particularly challenging due to discomfort around the topic.

Opting for the medical path would mean positioning our product behind healthcare practitioners, limiting its visibility, and essentially waiting for patients to seek it out actively. It's essential to recognize that most people don't proactively consult doctors for these intimate issues. On the other hand, choosing the wellness approach allows our company to cast a wider net, reaching a larger market and serving a more diverse range of users. I firmly believe that strictly adhering to the medical route might offer some ease but would likely cater to only about 20 percent of the potential user base.

This decision involves a trade-off between the convenience of operating in a medical space and the potential broader reach and impact achievable with a sexual wellness focus. To illustrate, I can point to a specific example: a medical device called Viberect. Despite its effectiveness, it remains relatively unknown because it operates purely in the medical realm, relying on urologists for awareness and accessibility.

At MysteryVibe, we're deeply involved in two main areas: first, crafting FDA Class 2 medical devices specifically designed to address a range of sexual health issues, and second, generating content that answers questions and kick-starts conversations around sexual wellness. Our medical devices are intricately designed to tackle concerns like erectile dysfunction, arousal disorders, peri- and postmenopausal symptoms, period pain, and postnatal pain. These devices leverage cutting-edge technologies to deliver precise vibrations to targeted areas.

We operate two distinct websites to cater to different needs: MysteryVibe, a customer-centric and pleasure-focused platform, and MySexMD, a doctor-centric site providing information for healthcare professionals. Our marketing approach draws parallels to condom marketing, emphasizing pleasure and enjoyment rather than clinical aspects to reach a broader audience less inclined to seek medical solutions actively.

In collaboration with doctors in the US and the UK, we identify topics that pose challenges for healthcare practitioners, research to assess the potential benefits of vibration, and kick-start developing prototypes. Through small trials and iterative processes based on user feedback, our devices evolve to a stage where they are both effective and safe for use.

Additionally, we engage in cohort studies to evaluate the real-world efficacy of our products.

I want to underscore the significance of making sexual wellness products accessible and enjoyable, steering away from framing them solely as solutions to clinical problems. This approach aims to diminish the stigma and shame associated with sexual health issues.

* * *

This chapter on women's sexual health illuminates the persistent challenges and emerging solutions within the realm of female sexual well-being. Central to the discussion is the recognition of women's sexual health as a crucial aspect of their overall well-being, historically neglected and shrouded in taboo. Through the innovative use of SexTech, including platforms like MakeLoveNotPorn, and Lioness, and apps like Rosy, there is a concerted effort to demystify female sexuality, providing women with the tools and knowledge to explore and enhance their sexual experiences. Moreover, these technological advancements empower women to understand their bodies better and address issues ranging from pleasure disparities to medical conditions like sexual dysfunction, highlighting a significant shift toward more inclusive and comprehensive sexual health education and support. The growing investment in SexTech and the increasing acknowledgment of the importance of female pleasure signify a promising trend toward achieving equity in sexual health and dismantling long-standing stigmas.

# Chapter 5
# Contraception

**FOR MONTHS, EMILY HAD BEEN DISMISSING THE** sharp cramps on her side as mere gas, echoing her mother's assurances that it was nothing serious. However, the pain progressively worsened, escalating to a point where she could no longer bear it. One excruciating night, the pain intensified so severely that, clutching her side, Emily convinced her mom to take her to the doctor. The next day, an ultrasound revealed a large ovarian cyst, looming ominously and threatening severe complications if it were to rupture. The discovery was alarming, and immediate action was necessary; a visit to the gynecologist was scheduled for the very next day, followed by an urgent surgical procedure set for later in the week to remove the cyst—a precaution to prevent the unbearable pain that would ensue if the cyst burst.

Navigating the adult world of gynecological health was a daunting prospect for Emily, compounded by her anxiety over personal judgments regarding her body. The vulnerability of having someone examine her so intimately was terrifying. She was particularly self-conscious about whether the doctors would judge her choice to shave or not to shave her pubic hair—a significant concern for a young woman who had only acquired this hair a few years earlier. Post-surgery, as Emily recovered, her doctor recommended birth control to prevent future cysts, which also had the added benefits of managing her acne and menstrual cramps. Although she had never envisioned herself taking birth control, especially since she identified as gay and saw no need for its contraceptive use, the medication proved beneficial. Emily's experience broadened her understanding of health and self-care, reshaping her approach to her body's needs and the medical decisions affecting her life. Since the surgery and starting the medication, she has not developed any new cysts, an outcome that brought relief and a newfound trust in her healthcare decisions.

The evolution of contraception is a narrative of innovation, societal shifts, and the quest for reproductive autonomy. In the early stages, options were rudimentary and often unsafe, relying on barrier methods like the condom, which has been in use in various forms for centuries, or on more unreliable methods such as withdrawal. The early twentieth century saw the development of diaphragms and cervical caps, which offered women more control but still required access to a healthcare provider for fitting. These methods, while revolutionary at the time, underscored the urgent need for more accessible and effective forms of contraception that women themselves could control.

The mid-twentieth century marked a turning point with the introduction of the birth control pill in 1960, a watershed moment in the history of contraception. For the first time, women could control their fertility through a simple daily oral medication. The pill's development was not just a scientific breakthrough but a catalyst for social change, enabling women to pursue higher education and careers, thereby altering traditional family structures and societal roles. However, the pill also sparked debates around morality, freedom, and women's rights, reflecting broader cultural tensions of the era.

Since then, the landscape of contraception has continued to diversify and expand, with the development of long-acting reversible contraceptives (LARCs) like intrauterine devices (IUDs) and implants, offering efficacy and convenience previously unimaginable. Today, research is focused not only on improving the safety and effectiveness of existing methods but also on expanding the range of options, including efforts to develop male contraceptives. This ongoing evolution of contraception mirrors the changing dynamics of society, where the demand for reproductive autonomy and gender equality continues to drive innovation and access in the field of reproductive health.

Women use birth control for a myriad of reasons that extend far beyond the primary aim of preventing pregnancy. One significant reason is to manage various medical conditions and menstrual-related issues, such as polycystic ovary syndrome (PCOS), endometriosis, and excessively heavy or painful periods. Hormonal contraceptives, such as the pill, the patch, or the ring, can regulate menstrual cycles, reduce the severity of menstrual cramps, and alleviate the symptoms of PCOS by regulating hormones.[47] Moreover, birth control methods like the hormonal IUD can significantly lessen menstrual flow and pain, providing relief for those with conditions like endometriosis, where the lining of the uterus grows outside of it, causing severe pain and menstrual irregularities.[48]

Beyond health management, birth control serves as a tool for women to exercise autonomy over their reproductive lives, enabling them to make choices about if or when to have children. This reproductive control can have profound impacts on a woman's ability to pursue educational and career goals without the interruption of unplanned pregnancies. It also allows couples and individuals to plan their families, ensuring that children are brought into environments where they are wanted and can be well cared for. The ability to control one's reproductive health is intrinsically linked to broader issues of gender equality, as it ensures women can participate fully in all aspects of society. Thus, birth control is a pivotal element not only in individual healthcare but in the broader context of social and economic empowerment for women.

Some women need or want nonhormonal birth control due to various reasons, including health-related issues, personal preferences, or religious beliefs. Health concerns such as sensitivity to hormones, increased risk of blood clots, or adverse side effects like mood changes from hormonal contraceptives can lead women to seek nonhormonal options. Personal preferences may include desiring a birth control method that doesn't interfere with the body's natural hormonal balance or wanting to avoid the potential systemic side effects associated with hormonal methods. Additionally, some women opt for nonhormonal birth control as it aligns more closely with their lifestyle, offering a more natural approach to family planning without the need for daily medication. Nonhormonal methods, such as copper IUDs, condoms, and fertility awareness-based methods, provide effective alternatives that cater to these diverse needs, allowing women to have control over their reproductive health in a way that best suits their individual circumstances.

Women's ability to access birth control is influenced by a myriad of factors, creating a landscape where the freedom to choose if, when, and how to use contraception is not uniformly available. Financial constraints, lack of insurance coverage, and high costs of some birth control methods can significantly limit access, especially for low-income women.[49] Geographic barriers, such as living in areas with limited healthcare facilities or in contraceptive deserts where the full range of contraceptive options is not readily available, further exacerbate the issue. Legal and policy restrictions, alongside cultural and societal stigmas, can also pose significant barriers, particularly in regions with conservative views on reproductive rights or where misinformation about contraception prevails. Moreover, the prescription requirement for certain methods introduces an additional hurdle, requiring women to navigate the healthcare system, which can be daunting due to time constraints, privacy concerns, and sometimes judgmental attitudes from healthcare providers. Despite these barriers, advancements in telehealth and policy efforts aimed at improving contraceptive equity are gradually expanding access, illustrating a growing recognition of birth control as a fundamental aspect of women's healthcare and autonomy.

The advent of birth control has played a pivotal role in transforming women's roles in society, marking a profound shift in the landscape of gender equality and personal autonomy. Before the widespread availability of contraceptives, women's lives were often dictated by the unrelenting cycle of childbirth and childrearing, limiting their opportunities for education and participation in the workforce. Birth control emerged as a liberating force, granting women the power to decide whether and when to have children, thereby opening new avenues for professional and personal development. This newfound control over their reproductive lives enabled women to pursue higher education, embark on careers, and contribute to economic growth and societal progress on an unprecedented scale. The ability to plan pregnancies meant that women could invest in their futures with greater confidence, breaking traditional gender roles and paving the way for a more inclusive and equitable society.

Planned Parenthood has been instrumental in the distribution and promotion of birth control, playing a crucial role in the reproductive rights movement. Founded by Margaret Sanger, a pioneering advocate for women's rights and contraception, Planned Parenthood began as a clinic offering birth control information and has since evolved into a nationwide network providing a wide range of reproductive health services. By making contraceptives more accessible and affordable, Planned Parenthood has helped countless women take control of their reproductive health, regardless of their socioeconomic status. The organization has also been at the forefront of advocacy efforts, fighting for the legal and social acceptance of birth control, and challenging policies and regulations that restrict access to contraceptives. Through education, outreach, and legal battles, Planned Parenthood has contributed significantly to the normalization and acceptance of birth control, empowering women to make informed choices about their bodies and futures.

The impact of birth control on women's roles in society, supported by organizations like Planned Parenthood, has been transformative. By promoting reproductive autonomy, birth control has not only enhanced women's personal freedom but has also contributed to societal advancements by enabling women to participate more fully in all aspects of life. The role of Planned Parenthood in distributing and advocating for birth control has been invaluable, ensuring that women across the nation have the resources and support they need to navigate their reproductive health. As we move forward, the continued availability and acceptance of birth control, championed by advocates and organizations dedicated to women's rights, will remain essential in the ongoing struggle for gender equality and the empowerment of women worldwide. And just as Planned Parenthood paved the way for the contraception revolution, so too do these FemTech startups.

## Sophia Yen, MD, MPH, Cofounder and CMO at Pandia Health

*Pandia Health is a women-founded, women-led, doctor-led birth control delivery company. Episode 9 aired May 11, 2020.*

### What does Pandia Health offer?

Pandia Health provides a convenient service where if you have a prescription, you can tell us where it's at, and provide your insurance information. We will deliver your birth control directly to your door every month or every three months, depending on what your insurance or doctor has approved. We also include free goodies and educational materials in every package, because we believe in empowering women with knowledge about their health options. For example, we educate about the effectiveness of generic medications and different types of emergency contraception.

Telehealth for birth control is critical because it addresses several barriers that women face in accessing contraception, especially in OB-GYN deserts—areas where there are few or no obstetricians/gynecologists. Many women live far from the nearest healthcare provider or cannot find time for an appointment due to busy schedules or lack of transportation. Telehealth simplifies this process by allowing women to receive birth control without needing to physically visit a doctor's office, ensuring continuous access to necessary reproductive healthcare.

### Is it safe for women to skip their period using hormonal birth control?

First, let's talk about the frequency of periods. Historically, women used to have around one-hundred periods in their lifetime. This was due to frequent pregnancies and extended periods of breastfeeding, which naturally suppressed menstruation. Now, the scenario has changed drastically. Modern women experience approximately 350 to 400 periods over their lifetime. This significant increase is due to a combination of factors, including fewer pregnancies, shorter durations of breastfeeding, and earlier onset of menstruation (now often around the age of twelve, compared to fifteen or sixteen in the past).

This change in menstrual frequency isn't without its implications. The increased number of periods presents several health risks, including a higher likelihood of developing anemia, particularly in menstruating women, and an increased risk of ovarian and endometrial cancers. The frequent fluctuation in hormones and the physical process of menstruation can also impact women's daily lives, causing discomfort, pain, and inconvenience.

Given these factors, it's worth considering making periods optional. This isn't just about convenience; it has tangible health benefits. By using birth control methods like the pill, patch, or ring, women can safely reduce the frequency of their periods. This approach not only decreases the risk of ovarian and endometrial cancers but also combats the leading cause of anemia in menstruating women. Furthermore, for women in demanding careers or those with active lifestyles, having control over their menstrual cycle can be empowering and beneficial for their overall quality of life. But these busy women need to remember to take their pills every day.

## Amanda French, Cofounder and Former CEO at Emme

*The Emme Smart Case and app is an integrated technology-enabled solution designed to safeguard the birth control experience and help reduce the rate of missed pills. Episode 93 aired February 24, 2021.*

**Tell us about birth control pill usage in the US.**

There are ten million women in the US on birth control pills at any given time, and 150 million women worldwide. The pill is the most common form of contraception and one of the most prescribed drugs, especially for teenage girls and women in their twenties. It's often their first prescription. This is their entry point into the healthcare system for tens of millions of women.

Unfortunately, though, nearly one out of ten people on the pill have an unplanned pregnancy each year, amounting to a million unplanned pregnancies. Most of these unplanned pregnancies are due to adherence challenges, i.e., forgetting to take their pill every day.

**What is Emme?**

We commercialized a smart pill case for birth control pill adherence. It's a small, sleek, connected case with Bluetooth capabilities and multiple sensors. It tracks when you have taken your pill and automatically syncs that data with our app. The real magic happens with the app because, for users of our product, we have data about their medication use, allowing our app to send smart and relevant reminders until the pill is taken.

Alarm fatigue is a common issue. People often think they'll remember to take their pill, but they end up ignoring constant reminders. Our system sends reminders only when you've missed your pills, making them much more relevant. You can customize these reminders, whether a text or push notification and receive up to three reminders. This personalized approach reduces missed pills by 80 percent.

In one of our recent studies, we found that our app helps people take the pill on time and provides valuable information. It answers questions like what to do if you miss a pill or whether you're on the right pill for your body. Our app offers details from the Centers for Disease Control and Prevention on what to do if you miss a pill and allows you to track symptoms and side effects. It provides a comprehensive view of your medication experience and aligns with our broader vision of driving innovation throughout the entire women's health journey. Our goal is to help women have an optimal contraception experience, even if that is realizing that the hormonal pill is not the best option for them.

## Saundra Pelletier, CEO at Evofem Biosciences

*Evofem Biosciences, Inc., focuses on commercializing innovative products to address unmet needs in women's sexual and reproductive health. Their product, Phexxi, offers a hormone-free option that allows women to maintain their natural vaginal pH, effectively preventing conception. Episode 61 aired November 9, 2020.*

### Why are nonhormonal birth controls important for women?

Statistics show that a staggering number of women, about twenty-one million in the United States, actively seek alternatives to hormonal birth control. One contributing factor may be the side effects they experience, such as weight gain, mood changes, and loss of libido. The need for nonhormonal options is not just a matter of comfort; it's about giving women control and choice regarding their reproductive health. Women should have the freedom to decide when and how to use contraception without compromising their well-being.

Nonhormonal methods like Phexxi cater to this need, providing an on-demand option that women can use only when necessary. This approach aligns perfectly with the ethos of empowering women by allowing them to make informed choices about their bodies without the daily commitment or systemic side effects of hormonal methods or risk of drug-drug interactions.

Moreover, nonhormonal methods are crucial for specific groups of women. For instance, breastfeeding mothers, women with contraindications to hormones (like a history of certain cancers), or those concerned about the long-term effects of hormonal therapies on their fertility, find immense value in products like Phexxi. It's about inclusivity in healthcare, ensuring every woman has access to a contraceptive method that aligns with her health needs, lifestyle, and preferences.

### What is the role of pH in fertility and contraception?

The vaginal environment's pH plays a crucial role in reproductive health. A typical vaginal pH is between 3.5 and 4.5, an acidic environment that naturally combats harmful bacteria. However, during intercourse, semen, which has a higher pH, can alter this balance, increasing the vaginal pH to around seven or eight. This shift is essential for sperm survival and it facilitates pregnancy. Our product, Phexxi, is designed to maintain the vagina's natural acidity even in the presence of semen, thus maintaining an environment that is inhospitable to sperm. This mechanism offers women a unique method of contraception that is both effective and respectful of their body's natural processes. It's exciting to see all the innovations in contraception outside of the pill including devices like the IUD.

## Jessica Grossman, MD, Former CEO at Medicines360

*Medicines360 is a nonprofit pharmaceutical organization prioritizing women over profit to ensure equitable access to medicines. Their product, Liletta, has significantly impacted expanding reproductive choices not only in the United States but also in low- and middle-income countries. Episode 56 aired October 21, 2020.*

### Tell us about Medicines360 mission and products.

Historically, hormonal intrauterine devices (IUDs) for contraception were prohibitively expensive, creating disparities in access. To address this, we secured funding from an anonymous donor in 2009 to develop an affordable hormonal IUD that maintained effectiveness, safety, and long-acting features. Our mission was rooted in addressing inequities in access to this essential contraceptive.

In our quest for a hormonal IUD, we discovered a product produced by a small pharmaceutical company in Liege, Belgium. Lacking the resources to bring it to the US, we initiated a significant phase-three, US study in 2009 to obtain FDA approval. Unlike conventional studies, we designed ours with equity, challenging contraception misconceptions. Our diverse study included women who had never given birth, those with high BMI (body mass index), and participants from various races and ethnicities. This approach resulted in FDA approval in 2015.

Despite being a nonprofit, we operated like a small startup, ensuring agility and speed. Our ongoing phase-three, clinical study involves twenty-nine active sites and spans ten years to comprehensively understand the hormonal IUD's long-term effectiveness. Our primary goals include women's empowerment, economic liberation, and reducing unintended pregnancies.

Our product, Liletta, is available in the US, and we have a co-marketing partnership with AbbVie. Between 2016 and 2021, over half a million units have been used, with approximately 260,000 units utilized in low-income clinics. We also hold rights to the product in low- and middle-income countries, which enables us to implement the Avibela Project in Africa. Registered in several African countries, including Zambia, Nigeria, Kenya, and Madagascar, our collaboration with NGO partners has introduced the method, with overwhelmingly positive feedback and high satisfaction rates, particularly in Madagascar. Research indicates that 60 percent of women adopting the hormonal IUD in Madagascar might not have chosen any contraception method otherwise, underscoring the initiative's significant impact on expanding reproductive choices. With IUDs being such a success story for women, we should now turn our attention to the process of inserting it into the uterus which has serious pain associated with it.

## Ikram Guerd, VP of Global Marketing at Aspivix

*Aspivix designed the first suction-cervical stabilizer, reducing pain and bleeding in IUD insertions and other gynecological procedures.*
*Episode 230 aired March 13, 2024.*

**How are intrauterine devices (IUDs) inserted into the uterus? Why is it painful?**

IUD insertion involves several steps to ensure the device is accurately placed within the uterus for effective contraception. The process begins with the opening of the vagina using a speculum, followed by the insertion of the IUD through the cervical canal into the uterus. A crucial part of this procedure involves using a tenaculum, an instrument designed to stabilize the cervix by grasping it, allowing the physician to accurately measure the uterus and facilitate the insertion of the IUD. The tenaculum, however, is a source of significant discomfort and pain for many women undergoing this procedure.

The tenaculum is a surgical instrument with a history of over a century. Invented initially to extract bullets from soldiers, its sharp, scissor-like appearance and function make it quite intimidating. Its design, comprising two sharp teeth, allows it to grasp and hold the cervix firmly, which can cause puncturing and subsequent bleeding, contributing to the pain experienced during IUD insertion.

Pain during IUD insertion varies among women but is notably significant due to the invasiveness of using the tenaculum. It's not merely about the pinch felt; for many, the experience can be deeply traumatic, leading to bleeding, dizziness, and in some cases, fainting. This pain is not a fleeting moment; it can have lingering effects, making the overall experience daunting for women seeking long-term contraception.

## Is women's pain during IUD insertion being taken seriously?

In the healthcare system, women's pain is often underestimated and not taken as seriously as it should be. There's a significant disconnect between the pain women express and how healthcare professionals perceive it. When women report pain, it's not uncommon for it to be downplayed, attributing it to women being too sensitive or too emotional. This bias against women's pain is a critical issue that needs addressing.

Pain management during IUD insertion is minimal at best. Typically, women might be advised to take an over-the-counter pain reliever like Advil before the procedure, but that's about it. The pain from the insertion process, significantly amplified using instruments like the tenaculum, is vastly underestimated. Often, women are not adequately warned about the potential intensity of the pain they might experience. There's a lack of comprehensive communication about what the procedure entails and its associated discomforts, possibly due to the fear of increasing anxiety or because the pain is unjustly minimized.

The dismissal or under-addressing of women's pain can partly be attributed to long-standing biases and stereotypes within the healthcare system. These biases include the belief that women are more prone to exaggerate their pain or that pain related to female-specific procedures is just something women should accept. This is deeply problematic because it leads to a lack of adequate pain management strategies and contributes to the perpetuation of the idea that women's health issues are not as critical or deserving of attention. It's a cycle that reinforces itself, keeping women's pain in the shadows and impeding progress toward more empathetic and effective healthcare practices for women.

Aspivix is tackling the issue of pain during IUD insertion head-on with our innovative device, the Carevix. This device is a significant departure from the traditional, painful methods using a tenaculum. The Carevix employs a gentle suction mechanism to stabilize the cervix without needing sharp, pinching claws. By creating a vacuum seal, it securely holds the cervix in place, allowing for more precise, less traumatic access during procedures such as IUD insertions, endometrial biopsies, and hysteroscopies.

* * *

The journey through the contraception chapter illuminates a pivotal narrative in women's health and empowerment, underscoring the profound impact that access to diverse contraceptive options has had on individual lives and society at large. The evolution of contraception from rudimentary barrier methods to sophisticated hormonal and nonhormonal options has not only expanded choices for women but also catalyzed shifts in societal roles and family structures. This transformation is not just about preventing unwanted pregnancies, it's also about enabling women to make strategic life choices, enhancing their autonomy over their health and affirming their roles in the workforce and education sectors. As we look forward, the continued innovation and accessibility in contraception promise to further refine and redefine the landscape of women's health, ensuring that every woman has the freedom and the means to make informed decisions about her body and her future.

# Chapter 6
# Fertility

**SABRINA HAD ALWAYS IMAGINED MOTHERHOOD** as part of her future, but the shadow of endometriosis loomed large over her dreams. Since her teenage years, she's been managing the pain and complications of her condition while also carrying a constant vigilance against pregnancy. Now, with her partner by her side and a deep yearning to start a family, she found herself in an ironic twist of fate—needing to figure out how to achieve the very thing she had spent so long trying to prevent. The reality of possibly not being able to conceive naturally due to her endometriosis was a bitter pill to swallow, adding layers of frustration and sadness to her already complex feelings about her body and fertility.

After a year of trying without success, their hopes dwindling with each passing month, Sabrina and her partner decided to consult a fertility clinic. The tests conducted there revealed something unexpected: Sabrina was severely deficient in vitamin D, a factor that might have been impeding her ability to conceive. Embarking on a regimen of high-dose vitamin D supplements, she approached this new phase with a mix of skepticism and hope. Remarkably, just four months later, Sabrina discovered she was pregnant. Relief and gratitude washed over her, tempered only by a tinge of frustration that such a simple solution had taken so long to uncover. While she was thankful for the medical intervention that ultimately helped her achieve her dream of pregnancy, she couldn't help but wish that her earlier healthcare providers had tested for such imbalances sooner, possibly sparing her months of unnecessary anguish.

Infertility, a condition that affects millions worldwide, is defined by the World Health Organization (WHO) as the failure to achieve a pregnancy after twelve months or more of regular unprotected sexual intercourse.[50] Its global impact is profound, with recent estimates suggesting that approximately 17.5 percent of adults globally experience some form of infertility, translating to one in six people facing challenges in conceiving. This widespread issue crosses cultural, racial, and socioeconomic boundaries, making it a critical concern for public health and individual well-being.[51] The condition poses significant challenges to population growth and demographic balance in various regions and highlights the need for accessible and effective fertility treatments and supportive policies around the globe.

A closer examination of infertility rates reveals notable differences across various regions and income levels, illustrating the complex interplay of genetic, environmental, and socioeconomic factors in fertility health. High-income countries tend to report slightly higher rates of infertility, attributed partly to the tendency of individuals in these countries to delay childbearing for educational, career, and personal reasons, which can reduce fertility potential over time. Conversely, in low- and middle-income countries, where access to fertility treatments is often limited, the rates of infertility are slightly lower but still significant, reflecting the global nature of this issue. Additionally, environmental factors, such as pollution and exposure to toxins, along with lifestyle choices, such as smoking and obesity, contribute to the varying rates of infertility observed across different regions and income groups.[52]

The journey through infertility often brings with it not just medical challenges, but deep emotional and financial burdens as well. Couples and individuals grappling with infertility may experience a roller coaster of hope and disappointment, often accompanied by stigma and isolation, impacting their mental health and emotional resilience. Financially, the situation can be just as daunting, with the high costs of fertility treatments such as in vitro fertilization (IVF) placing a substantial strain on personal finances. These treatments, often not covered by insurance, can lead to significant debt, with many having to make difficult choices about pursuing their dream of parenthood. The intersection of emotional and financial stress underscores the complexity of infertility, highlighting the need for comprehensive support systems that address both the medical and socio-economic aspects of this challenging journey.

The rise in global infertility rates can be attributed to a confluence of lifestyle changes and environmental factors that have altered the reproductive landscape. Modern lifestyles, characterized by high stress, poor diet, obesity, and increased exposure to pollutants, have been linked to decreased fertility in both men and women.[53] Stress, in particular, has been shown to affect hormonal balance, while obesity can lead to ovulatory disorders.[54,55] Environmental factors, such as exposure to chemicals and toxins found in pesticides, plastics, and industrial pollutants, have been associated with reduced sperm quality in men and ovulatory disorders in women.[56] These lifestyle and environmental shifts, compounded by a global trend toward delayed childbearing for reasons ranging from career progression to financial stability, underscore the multifaceted causes behind the increasing rates of infertility observed worldwide.

Age plays a critical role in female fertility, with a noticeable decline beginning in the late twenties and accelerating after the age of thirty-five. By the age of forty, the chances of natural conception drop significantly, with studies showing that fertility decreases by as much as half compared to women in their early twenties.[57] This age-related decline in fertility is due to both a decrease in the quantity and quality of a woman's eggs.[58] Medical conditions further exacerbate the challenge of infertility; polycystic ovary syndrome (PCOS) and endometriosis are prominent examples that affect a significant number of women of reproductive age. PCOS, marked by hormonal imbalances that interfere with ovulation, is a leading cause of female infertility.[59] Endometriosis, where endometrial tissue grows outside the uterus, can lead to fallopian tube obstruction and infertility.[60] Male-factor infertility, accounting for approximately one-third of infertility cases, is characterized by issues with sperm production, function, or delivery, highlighting the importance of addressing both partners in infertility assessments and treatments.[61] These factors illuminate the complex interplay between age, health conditions, and modern life in the rising infertility rates.

Fertility treatments offer a beacon of hope for many struggling with infertility, spanning a wide array of options from medication to assist in ovulation to advanced assisted reproductive technologies (ART) such as

IVF and intracytoplasmic sperm injection (ICSI). Medications like clomiphene citrate or gonadotropins are often the first line of treatment to stimulate ovulation in women with disorders such as PCOS. For more complex cases, ARTs, including IVF, where eggs are fertilized outside the body and then implanted into the uterus, and ICSI, a technique where a single sperm is injected directly into an egg, offer alternative paths to conception. These technologies have revolutionized fertility treatment, offering solutions even in cases of severe male infertility or fallopian tube damage.

However, these treatments come with their own set of challenges and costs. Success rates vary widely depending on factors like age, the specific infertility diagnosis, and the clinic chosen for treatment. For instance, IVF success rates decrease significantly with the patient's age, with younger women generally experiencing higher success rates. The financial burden of these treatments can also be considerable, often exceeding tens of thousands of dollars per treatment cycle, with many requiring multiple cycles to achieve pregnancy. Despite these obstacles, innovations in fertility technology continue to advance the field. Egg freezing offers women the opportunity to preserve their fertility until they are ready to start a family. At the same time, genetic screening of embryos can increase the likelihood of a healthy pregnancy, addressing genetic diseases before pregnancy begins. These advancements represent cutting-edge fertility treatment, aimed at not only improving success rates but also extending the window of fertility for individuals and couples around the world.

The trend of companies offering fertility benefits to employees has gained momentum as organizations recognize the value of supporting diverse family-building paths for their workforce. Notable companies across various industries, including tech giants like Google and Facebook, have led the way by implementing comprehensive fertility benefits, covering treatments from IVF to egg freezing. These initiatives have positively impacted employee retention and satisfaction, with staff members expressing gratitude for the support in their personal family-planning journeys. Moreover, fertility benefits play a crucial role in promoting diversity, equity, and inclusion in the workplace by acknowledging and addressing the needs of LGBTQIA+ employees, single parents, and those facing medical challenges related to fertility. By offering such benefits, companies send a strong message of inclusivity and commitment to supporting their employees' well-being and life choices, enhancing their reputation as desirable places to work.

The future of fertility technology is poised for groundbreaking advancements, with emerging technologies in the field of reproductive health promising to revolutionize how fertility care is delivered. Innovations such as artificial intelligence (AI) for improved embryo selection, noninvasive genetic screening, and advancements in stem cell research can make fertility treatments more accessible, effective, and personalized. These technologies could significantly reduce costs and increase success rates, making the dream of parenthood a reality for a broader range of individuals and couples. However, as we navigate this promising future, ethical considerations around genetic editing, embryo selection, and the implications of increasingly personalized fertility treatment plans must be carefully addressed. The focus will be on balancing the benefits of these innovations with ethical standards and ensuring equitable access to these advanced reproductive technologies.

Fertility is one of the most popular sectors of women's health for innovation. There are a disproportionate number of male founders in fertility compared to the other women's health verticals. It could be safe to assume that this is because of their equal involvement in the conception process and an equal variable during infertility. Here we explore innovators from around the world improving the fertility journey.

## Amy Beckley, PhD, Founder and CEO at Proov

*Proov is a developer of urine progesterone test strips designed to track ovulation and diagnose hormonal imbalances at home.*
*Episode 151 aired January 27, 2022.*

### Why did you start Proov?

Starting Proov was driven by a deeply personal journey and the recognition of a significant gap in women's healthcare. My own struggles with infertility and recurrent miscarriage revealed a stark reality: The existing medical system often leaves women with more questions than answers, especially when it comes to understanding their own bodies. As a scientist with a PhD in pharmacology, I refused to accept unexplained infertility as an answer. The journey through IVF, and the miracle of eventually having my children, only intensified my commitment to empower other women. I knew there had to be a better way to provide insights into women's reproductive health.

Fertility treatments are considered elective procedures so are not covered by insurance. Clinical definitions of infertility often require attempting for twelve or more months, creating challenges for those seeking assistance before reaching that timeframe. Empowering doctors with better resources, like the Proov tool, could improve conversations and outcomes.

### What does Proov offer?

We are a pioneering company specializing in at-home hormone testing, particularly focusing on progesterone, a crucial hormone for fertility and overall reproductive health. Our flagship product is an innovative at-home test that measures the metabolites of progesterone in urine, providing crucial information about a woman's ovulation quality and her body's readiness for pregnancy.

During IVF, progesterone is crucial for supporting the uterine lining after embryo transfer. The absence of sufficient progesterone can lead to pregnancy losses. While progesterone is standard in IVF cycles, there's limited research on its impact in natural cycles due to funding biases favoring IVF-related studies. My personal experience revealed that my insufficient progesterone levels were what was causing my infertility. Once I supplemented progesterone, I was able to conceive and carry to term successfully. I wanted women to discover these potential easy fixes without having to go through IVF. Because once you have created the right environment for fertilization and implantation, you may just need to time it right.

## Kristina Cahojova, Founder and CEO at Kegg

*Kegg is a developer of a fertility-tracking device designed to monitor vaginal fluid. The company's device helps pinpoint the fertile window and ovulation up to a week in advance by detecting changes in cervical fluids. Episode 11 aired May 18, 2020.*

### What is cervical fluid and what is its role in female health?

Cervical fluid is a crucial element in understanding women's fertility and health, produced by the cervix to facilitate or prevent sperm from entering the uterus. Its consistency and composition change throughout the menstrual cycle in response to hormonal fluctuations. It serves multiple purposes: facilitating sperm movement during fertile periods, protecting against infections, and acting as a natural barrier. Contrary to common misconceptions, cervical fluid, rather than the swiftness of sperm, determines which sperm can enter the reproductive system. This fluid undergoes a transformation that can also thicken under the influence of certain contraceptives like IUDs and birth control pills to prevent conception. Despite its importance, assessing cervical fluid has been challenging outside laboratory environments until recent advancements. This company has pioneered making vaginal health more accessible through their product, kegg, which analyzes cervical fluid changes via electrolyte measurements. While primarily aiding conception efforts, kegg also promotes pelvic floor health. With over 25,000 American couples benefiting in just two years, the company's data collection on cervical fluid is poised to revolutionize understanding in this field.

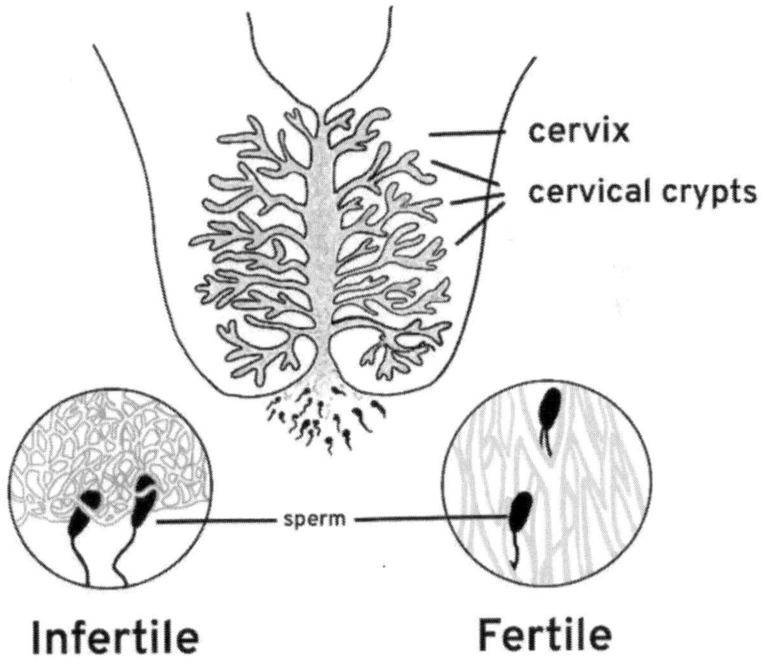


*Figure 10: The cervical crypts are responsible for creating cervical fluid which can either support or hinder the transport of sperm into the uterus.*

### What is kegg and how does it work?

Kegg is a fertility-monitoring device designed to help women understand their fertility by measuring changes in their cervical fluid. It operates on the principle of electrical impedance, utilizing gold-plated sensors to detect the unique electrolyte levels present in cervical fluid throughout different menstrual cycle stages. By inserting kegg into the vagina for just two minutes a day, the device collects data on the cervical fluid's electrolyte composition, which varies according to hormonal changes and fertility status.

Women can use kegg to identify their fertile window, the period when they are most likely to conceive. The device vibrates to guide users through a pelvic floor exercise during measurement, enhancing user experience and promoting pelvic health. After measurement, kegg wirelessly transmits the data to a companion app that analyzes and presents the user with insights into their fertility status, indicating the onset of the fertile window.

Kegg has been instrumental for couples trying to conceive, offering a user-friendly, noninvasive method to track fertility. Once the window of fertility is identified using kegg, couples can use other FemTech products that support the fertilization process.

## Maureen Brown, Cofounder and CEO at Mosie Baby

*The Mosie Baby Kit is a groundbreaking at-home insemination kit featuring the patented Mosie syringe. Episode 18 aired June 10, 2020.*

### What is Mosie Baby, and why did you start it?

My husband and I faced challenges conceiving our first child, leading us to start Mosie Baby. After two and a half years of unaided attempts and a diagnosis of unexplained infertility, we felt frustrated with the lack of specific solutions. Mosie Baby offers an at-home insemination method, specifically intra-cervical insemination (ICI), addressing the need we identified during our own journey. Designed for user experience, Mosie Baby provides helpful instructions, a supportive community, and an empowering way for individuals to create a baby at home on their own terms.

Mosie Baby is the evolved version of the traditional turkey baster. Recognizing the awkwardness and inefficiencies of existing methods, we designed a product that feels familiar, resembling a tampon. By mimicking

Mother Nature's design, including a slit opening similar to a man's penis, Mosie Baby ensures a more natural and efficient insemination process.

The Mosie Baby Kit includes two syringes, educational instructions, and collection cups for partners or donors. The process is straightforward: collect the sperm in the cup, suck up the sample into the syringe, insert it into the vagina, and push the sample in. This simple and straightforward approach makes Mosie Baby accessible for users seeking an effective at-home insemination solution. Especially considering this nearly identical procedure in a medical office costs patients between $300 and $1000 without insurance.

### How does the cervix change during the fertility window?

The cervix, a remarkable and often underrated component of the female reproductive system, undergoes significant changes throughout a woman's menstrual cycle, serving as a critical indicator of fertility. Its position, texture, and openness of its os (the opening to the uterus that connects the uterus to the vagina) alter in response to hormonal fluctuations, providing valuable cues for those tracking fertility for conception purposes. For example, during ovulation, the cervix typically becomes softer, sits higher in the vagina, and opens slightly to facilitate the passage of sperm. Conversely, it is firmer, lower, and closed at less fertile times. This dynamic nature of the cervix not only aids in the timing of intercourse for couples trying to conceive but also plays a protective role by acting as a barrier to the uterus, guarding against infections and facilitating the movement of sperm to the egg. Understanding these changes can empower women to become more attuned to their bodies and fertility, offering a natural method of family planning.

Mosie Baby provides a product to consumers at an accessible and affordable price before having to experience procedures in the doctor's office. I know many companies are creating exciting innovations in the fertility space if a woman does need additional support to become pregnant.

## Kathy Lee-Sepsick, MBA, Founder and CEO at Femasys

*Femasys's mission is to address underserved areas in women's health and pioneer innovations that are less invasive and more cost-effective than current practices. This encompasses advancements in contraception, fertility solutions, and biopsy products. Episode 146 aired December 20, 2021.*

## Tell us about the biology of fallopian tubes.

The fallopian tubes are fascinating and crucial components of the female reproductive system. They play a pivotal role in fertility and reproductive health. Biologically, the fallopian tubes are narrow, tubular structures connecting the ovaries to the uterus. They are about the size of spaghetti, approximately one to two millimeters in diameter at the opening, and they are where natural conception occurs.

The primary function of the fallopian tubes is to transport the ovum, or egg, from the ovaries to the uterus. During ovulation, the ovum is released from the ovary and enters the fallopian tube, where it may encounter sperm if conception is to occur. The tubes are lined with cilia, tiny hair-like structures that help move the ovum along the tube toward the uterus.

Fallopian tubes can be affected by various health conditions. For instance, blockages in the tubes, often resulting from infections such as pelvic inflammatory disease, can lead to challenges in conception. These blockages can prevent sperm from reaching the egg or stop the fertilized egg from reaching the uterus, leading to infertility or ectopic pregnancies. Interestingly, many women with blocked fallopian tubes may not exhibit symptoms, making diagnostic tests crucial for understanding fertility issues.

## What products has Femasys developed and what do they do?

We've developed several innovative products focusing on reproductive health, with each designed to address specific needs in women's healthcare. Our primary products are FemBloc, FemaSeed, FemVue, and FemCerv.

FemBloc is our flagship product, a permanent birth control option that offers a nonsurgical alternative to traditional tubal ligation. FemBloc works by delivering a biopolymer into the fallopian tubes, which then solidifies, ultimately triggering a wound-healing response creating a blockage, preventing pregnancy. This biopolymer is designed to be safe and natural, degrading over time and leaving behind tissue in-growth to maintain the blockage. It's a breakthrough in providing women with a less invasive, safer permanent contraception method.

FemaSeed is our latest innovation, targeting the front end of infertility treatments. FemaSeed is a device that delivers sperm directly to the fallopian tubes, optimizing the chances of natural conception. This approach is more directed and efficient compared to traditional intrauterine insemination, which can be undirected and less effective. It can also serve as a first step prior to expensive and invasive in vitro fertilization.

FemVue is a product that revolutionizes how physicians evaluate the health of fallopian tubes, which is essential prior to FemaSeed or any other infertility treatment. Traditionally, this process required a radiology appointment for an HSG (hysterosalpingogram), which uses X-rays and radiopaque dye. FemVue, on the other hand, uses a natural saline and air contrast that can be visualized with ultrasound. This method is far less invasive, doesn't require radiation, and can be performed in the comfort of the gynecologist's office.

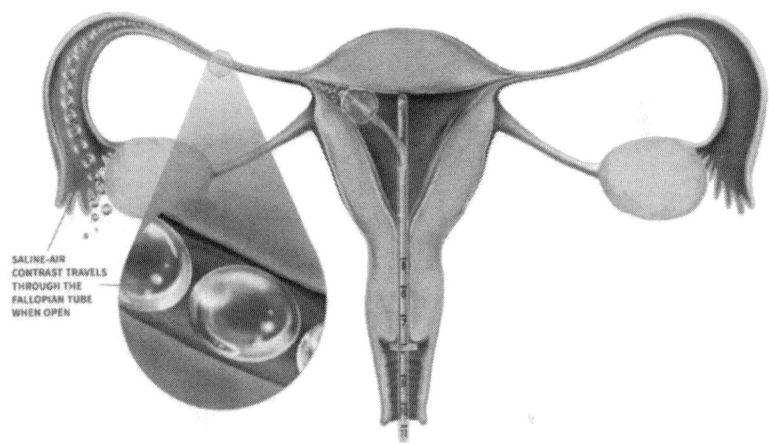


*Figure 11: Femasys's FemVue product enables visualization of the fallopian tubes and assists physicians in identifying potential blocks that may be causing infertility.*

FemCerv was developed as an advanced endocervical sampler for early detection of cervical cancer. Unlike traditional methods which can be suboptimal and uncomfortable, our device is designed to be gentle and efficient in sampling tissue for laboratory analysis. This advancement is significant in improving the diagnostic process for cervical cancer, making it less daunting for women.

Each of these products represents our commitment to enhancing women's healthcare experiences, focusing on safety, convenience, and efficacy. We're dedicated to transforming the landscape of gynecological care, offering more empowering choices for women globally. The advancements being made to the fertility industry are impressive, especially with the rise of artificial intelligence supporting clinical decisions.

## Ula Sankowska, Cofounder and CEO at MIM Fertility

*MIM Fertility employs AI to enhance the fertility journey and reproductive health. By leveraging a combination of AI software, advanced machine learning, and physician collaboration, their goal is to improve fertility treatments ultimately resulting in better outcomes.*
*Episode 218 aired September 27, 2023.*

### How does MIM Fertility's software work?

MIM Fertility's software represents a fusion of advanced machine learning, imaging solutions, and data-mining algorithms, integrated with the clinical expertise of reproductive medicine. Our primary goal is to empower doctors and patients, enhancing their ability to make well-informed decisions about fertility treatments.

Let's take a closer look at our software. First, we have EmbryoAid, designed for embryologists working in IVF labs. This tool utilizes advanced, computer-vision algorithms to assess and score embryos. The process is simple: An embryologist takes an image of an embryo and uploads it to our platform. Within seconds, EmbryoAid delivers a detailed report, scoring the embryo based on its potential for successful implantation. This decision-support tool effectively acts as a council of expert embryologists, deciding which embryo to transfer.

Another of our innovations is FolliScan, which aids ultrasonographers in fertility diagnosis. Using ultrasound, FolliScan identifies, counts, and measures follicles in a woman's ovaries. This process is crucial in determining a woman's fertility status and in monitoring the growth of follicles during IVF treatments. By automating and standardizing this process, FolliScan speeds up the examination and reduces human error, providing more accurate and consistent results.

Our software aims to bring precision and standardization to the IVF process. It's about seamlessly integrating technology into the workflow, enhancing the capabilities of fertility professionals, and ultimately improving patient outcomes.

## How will AI change fertility treatment in the future?

AI is set to revolutionize fertility treatment, opening new doors to what we can achieve in reproductive medicine. At the core of this transformation is AI's ability to process vast amounts of data with precision and speed, surpassing human capabilities in identifying patterns and making predictions.

First, AI will enhance the personalization of fertility treatments. By analyzing individual patient data, AI can tailor treatment protocols to each patient's specific needs, increasing the chances of success. This personalized approach is crucial because each fertility journey is unique, and what works for one patient may not work for another.

Second, AI will significantly improve the accuracy and efficiency of diagnosing fertility issues. It will provide more precise assessments of factors like ovarian reserve, sperm quality, and embryo development. This precision will enable us to make more informed decisions about treatment strategies, reducing the time, emotional stress, and financial burden typically associated with fertility treatments.

Furthermore, AI will democratize access to fertility care. By automating and standardizing many aspects of the fertility process, AI can help reduce costs and make these treatments more accessible to a broader range of patients. This aspect is particularly crucial because fertility care is often seen as a luxury. Still, with AI, it can become more of a standard healthcare service available to all who need it.

In terms of research and development, AI will accelerate the pace of discovery in fertility medicine. By analyzing data from thousands of fertility treatments, AI can uncover new insights into factors affecting fertility, leading to novel treatment methods and drugs.

Last, AI will play a pivotal role in genetic screening and embryo selection, enhancing the chances of a healthy pregnancy. With AI's ability to analyze complex genetic data, we can improve the embryo selection process, reducing the risk of genetic diseases and increasing the likelihood of successful implantation and pregnancy.

AI will be a game-changer in fertility treatment. It will usher in an era of more personalized, accurate, and accessible fertility care, helping countless individuals and couples realize their dreams of parenthood, especially as we continue to learn about all the factors that are influencing fertility like new research that shows the vaginal microbiome may have a more critical role than we thought.

## Gabriela Gutiérrez, PhD, Founder at Microgenesis

*Microgenesis conducts at-home functional microbiome tests for the intestinal and vaginal microbiome. Following the completion of the test, a restoration program is designed to address this imbalance and promote fertility. Episode 80 aired January 11, 2021.*

### What role does the vaginal microbiome play in fertility?

An imbalance or dysbiosis in the vaginal microbiome can lead to various issues, including infections, inflammation, and complications in conception and maintaining a healthy pregnancy.

In the context of fertility, a healthy vaginal microbiome is essential for creating a favorable environment for sperm survival and facilitating successful conception. Certain bacteria in the vaginal microbiome can impact the pH level of the vagina, making it more or less hospitable to sperm. A more acidic environment, for instance, can be hostile to sperm, reducing their viability and mobility, which in turn can affect fertilization.

Furthermore, an imbalanced vaginal microbiome can contribute to conditions like bacterial vaginosis, which has been linked to increased risks of miscarriage, preterm birth, and other pregnancy-related complications. This highlights the importance of maintaining a healthy vaginal microbiome not only for conception but also for the health of the pregnancy and the baby.

As a scientist focusing on reproductive immunology, I'm deeply interested in how the immune responses triggered by the microbiome affect fertility. Our research at Microgenesis is exploring the connections between the vaginal and gut microbiomes and their collective impact on reproductive health. By understanding these complex interactions, we aim to develop more effective, noninvasive treatments to enhance fertility and overall women's health.

### What is the science behind Microgenesis, and what are your results thus far?

The science behind Microgenesis is rooted in understanding the intricate relationship between the human microbiome—specifically the gut microbiome—and female fertility. Our approach is based on the concept that the gut microbiome plays a pivotal role in overall health, including reproductive health. The key lies in the microorganisms in our gut and how they influence bodily processes, including the immune system and hormonal balance, which are crucial for fertility.

Our research discovered that specific imbalances (dysbiosis) in the gut microbiome can lead to systemic inflammation and immune responses that adversely affect a woman's reproductive health. This can manifest as difficulties in conceiving, recurrent miscarriages, or complications during pregnancy. Identifying specific microorganisms lacking or overrepresented in the gut can create personalized probiotic treatments to restore balance and improve reproductive health.

We focus on noninvasive testing methods, including blood tests, saliva tests, and vaginal swabs, to assess various markers related to the gut microbiome and its impact on fertility. Based on these assessments, we tailor a regimen of probiotics and nutraceuticals (supplements designed to address nutritional deficiencies and enhance gut health).

Our results so far have been quite promising. In our clinical studies, we have included women who have had multiple unsuccessful IVF attempts. These are often seen as the most challenging fertility cases. Remarkably, we've seen a high rate of successful pregnancies following our Microgenesis treatment. In one study, around 75 percent of the women were able to conceive within six months after undergoing our treatment protocol. Moreover, 60 percent of these pregnancies were carried to term, resulting in the birth of healthy babies.

These outcomes demonstrate our approach's effectiveness in enhancing fertility and underscore the significance of gut health in overall reproductive wellness. By addressing underlying issues related to the microbiome, we can open new avenues for women struggling with fertility challenges, offering them hope and a more natural path to achieving pregnancy. We are excited to help ease the process of discovering why women may struggle to get pregnant because the fertility treatment process can be filled with questions and anxiety.

## Catherine Hendy, Cofounder at Elanza

*Elanza Wellness is a behavioral health coaching platform that recognizes the importance of prioritizing mental health throughout fertility treatments to reduce stress and improve outcomes. Episode 113 aired May 5, 2021.*

## How does stress affect fertility?

Stress has a profound impact on women's fertility, rooted in the biological mechanisms of our bodies. When we experience stress, particularly chronic stress, it triggers a cascade of hormonal reactions that can influence our reproductive system. The stress response involves our brain's hypothalamic-pituitary-adrenal (HPA) axis, which regulates stress hormones like cortisol. These hormones can affect the balance of reproductive hormones, potentially leading to irregular menstrual cycles, ovulation issues, and even impacting egg quality and fertility. It's a fascinating, though concerning, illustration of how closely our emotional state is linked to our physical well-being.

Fertility treatment itself can be a significant source of stress, which paradoxically can impact the very outcomes it aims to improve. The reasons are manifold. First, the process is inherently emotional and deeply personal, often embarked upon after a challenging journey of trying to conceive naturally. There's a profound sense of vulnerability in seeking help for something closely tied to one's identity and hopes for the future. Second, while medically necessary, the clinical environment and processes can feel impersonal and daunting, adding to the emotional burden. Additionally, the financial aspect of fertility treatments, which can be considerable and not always covered by insurance, compounds the stress, creating a cycle that's hard to break free from.

The stress around fertility treatments is not just about the treatments themselves but also about the surrounding circumstances, including societal pressures, the ticking of the biological clock, and the isolation that can come from undergoing such a personal journey. It underscores the necessity for a holistic approach to fertility care, one that addresses not just the physical aspects but also the emotional and psychological needs of individuals and couples navigating this path. This is why platforms like Elanza are stepping in to fill the gap, offering support that encompasses the whole person, not just their reproductive organs.

## What is Elanza, and why did you start it?

Elanza is a digital behavioral health coaching platform specifically designed for fertility patients. It was born out of personal experiences and the realization that fertility journeys, whether assisted or unassisted, are about more than just clinical treatments. My cofounder and I both underwent fertility treatments, including egg freezing, and realized through our experiences and conversations with peers that there was a significant gap in holistic care. We saw a need for support addressing the emotional, mental, and lifestyle aspects of fertility, beyond the clinical procedures.

Elanza aims to fill this gap by providing comprehensive support that considers the patient's entire well-being. It's built on the understanding that stress, lifestyle, and emotional health can tangibly impact fertility outcomes. We've collaborated with nearly thirty fertility experts worldwide, including doctors, scientists, and anthropologists, to gather insights and data that guide our platform's development.

The platform is designed to offer personalized, transformational journeys through fertility treatment, focusing on improving the odds of concepttion and pregnancy. It also aims to build resilience in patients facing the emotional and physical challenges of fertility struggles. By partnering with fertility clinics, Elanza integrates into existing workflows, offering additional support without overburdening clinic staff.

The inception of Elanza was driven by the desire to empower individuals on their fertility journeys, providing them with the tools and support needed to navigate the complex emotional and physical landscape of fertility treatments. We aim to improve the fertility experience, making it more holistic, supportive, and patient-centered. We know that women need every kind of support possible when on the journey to becoming mothers, including nutritional support.

* * *

In the illuminating exploration of fertility within the modern health paradigm, the narrative highlights the profound complexities and emotional intricacies of reproductive challenges. With an estimated 17.5 percent of adults globally grappling with infertility, this pervasive issue transcends cultural, socioeconomic, and geographic boundaries, underscoring a universal need for innovative and accessible fertility solutions.[62] This chapter delves into scientific advancements and technological innovations, such as AI-enhanced fertility treatments and at-home testing kits, which promise to democratize and personalize reproductive healthcare. It calls for a more integrated approach to fertility, blending emotional support and advanced medical treatments to assist countless individuals in realizing their dreams of parenthood.

# Chapter 7
# Pregnancy

**PREGNANCY MARKS THE BEGINNING** of a transformative journey where a woman's body nurtures and grows a fetus until birth. It typically spans around forty weeks from the last menstrual period, divided into three trimesters, each with its distinct developmental milestones for the fetus. The first trimester is crucial for the development of major organs, the second sees the growth and refinement of these structures, and the third prepares the fetus for birth. Interestingly, pregnancy is calculated from the first day of the last menstrual period, effectively including two weeks when the woman is not yet pregnant. It highlights the traditional method's lack of precision yet continued relevance in tracking pregnancy progression.

The physiological changes a woman undergoes during pregnancy are profound and varied, affecting nearly every system in the body. For instance, blood volume increases significantly to support the growing fetus, while hormonal changes can affect everything from metabolism to fluid retention.[63]

Pregnancy outcomes and experiences can vary widely among different populations, influenced by factors such as access to healthcare, socioeconomic status, and preexisting health conditions. For example, the Centers for Disease Control and Prevention (CDC) reports disparities in maternal and infant health outcomes, with certain groups experiencing higher rates of complications and mortality with Black and Indigenous women in the United States dying at rates three and two times higher than White women, respectively.[64,65] These disparities point to the need for a more equitable healthcare system that can provide tailored, comprehensive care to all pregnant women, ensuring both they and their babies have the best possible start.

Through the ages, childbirth has evolved significantly from a solely natural process to one that can be medically assisted, reflecting changes in societal attitudes, medical knowledge, and technology. In ancient times, childbirth was a mysterious and dangerous process, with high rates of maternal and infant mortality. The development of the human pelvis and increased brain size over millions of years made human childbirth more complex and riskier than other mammals.[66] These evolutionary changes necessitated assistance during childbirth, giving rise to the role of midwives who used herbal remedies and traditional techniques to aid women through labor.

The practice of midwifery, deeply rooted in communities, was passed down through generations, becoming an essential part of childbirth. Midwives were not just birth attendants; they were key figures in their communities, providing support, knowledge, and care to women before, during, and after birth. Midwives assisted women of all classes, including the wealthy and lower working-class women. However, the medicalization of childbirth in the nineteenth and twentieth centuries shifted the birthing process from home to hospital settings, with 88 percent of births occurring in hospitals by the 1950s, changing the role of midwives and increasing the use of interventions like cesarean sections.[67] While reducing certain risks associated with childbirth, this transition introduced new debates about the balance between natural and medicalized birthing processes, highlighting the need for a model of care that respects women's choices while ensuring safety.

Today, childbirth practices vary globally, influenced by cultural beliefs, medical practices, and access to healthcare. The increase in cesarean section rates, for example, reflects both advancements in medical interventions and concerns about their overuse. Similarly, the resurgence of interest in midwifery and natural birthing practices underscores a desire for more personalized, less interventionist childbirth experiences. As we continue to navigate the complexities of childbirth, we aim to ensure that all women have access to safe, respectful, and high-quality care, honoring their needs and preferences.

Miscarriage, the loss of a pregnancy before twenty weeks, is a common yet often silently borne experience, with estimates suggesting that about one in eight known pregnancies end in miscarriage.[68] Most miscarriages occur due to chromosomal abnormalities in the fetus, leading to a natural cessation of pregnancy.[69] Miscarriages are most common within the first trimester, with 80 percent of all miscarriages occurring within the first twelve weeks.[70] Despite its prevalence, miscarriage is frequently shrouded in silence and stigma, leaving many to navigate their grief and confusion without adequate support or understanding. This lack of open discussion contributes to misconceptions and isolation for those affected, underscoring the need for more awareness and compassionate care.

Efforts to demystify and destigmatize miscarriage have gained momentum, with more people sharing their experiences and advocating for better care and understanding. Such openness is crucial in changing perceptions and providing community and support for those affected. Additionally, ongoing research into the causes and prevention of miscarriage holds promise for reducing its incidence and improving care for those who experience it. As society becomes more open in discussing miscarriage, the hope is that those affected will feel less isolated and more supported in their journeys.

Pregnancy, while a natural process, is not without risks. Complications such as gestational diabetes and preeclampsia can significantly impact the health of both the mother and the fetus. Gestational diabetes, which affects how the cells use sugar, can lead to macrosomia. In this condition, the baby grows too large, increasing the risk of injuries during birth and the likelihood of a cesarean section. Preeclampsia, characterized by high blood pressure and signs of organ damage, can lead to severe complications if not managed promptly. There is no cure for preeclampsia besides preterm birth, highlighting the importance of regular prenatal monitoring.

Mental health challenges also pose significant risks during and after pregnancy. Research suggests that pregnancy complications increase the likelihood of postpartum depression. Conditions like depression and anxiety can have profound effects on the well-being of the mother, affecting her ability to care for herself and her baby. Despite being common, with postpartum depression affecting up to one in seven women, these conditions often go unrecognized and untreated, due to stigma and a lack of awareness among healthcare providers and patients alike.[71] This underscores the need for comprehensive screening and support systems to address mental health during pregnancy and the postpartum period.

The physical complications of pregnancy, such as hyperemesis gravidarum and placenta previa, further complicate the landscape of prenatal care. Hyperemesis gravidarum, an extreme form of morning sickness, can lead to dehydration and weight loss, requiring hospitalization in severe cases. Placenta previa, where the placenta covers the cervix, can cause severe bleeding during pregnancy and delivery, necessitating careful monitoring and possibly a cesarean section for delivery. These examples illustrate the complex interplay of factors affecting pregnancy outcomes, emphasizing the importance of personalized, comprehensive prenatal care.

Cesarean sections, surgical procedures to deliver a baby through the mother's abdomen, have become increasingly common, now accounting for more than one in five childbirths globally.[72] The rate of cesarean sections varies depending on location. For example, in Latin America, the rate is 43 percent, while in sub-Saharan Africa, it is only 5 percent.[73] This may indicate an accessibility issue depending on what part of the world someone is in. Ultimately, cesarean section rates have tripled from 7 percent in the 1990s to 21 percent today.[74] This rise reflects both the life-saving potential of cesarean sections in complicated deliveries and concerns about their overuse. In certain situations, such as abnormal fetal heart rate or the baby's position, a cesarean section is essential for the safety of the mother and baby. However, the increasing rate of elective cesarean sections, chosen without a medical indication, has sparked debate about the balance between medical necessity and preference.

Efforts to address the rising cesarean section rates focus on enhancing access to evidence-based prenatal care, promoting understanding of the natural birth process, and supporting women in making informed choices about their childbirth experiences. Reducing unnecessary cesarean sections and promoting safe, respectful maternity care practices can help ensure that both mothers and babies have the best possible health outcomes, aligning with global health recommendations and respecting women's autonomy in childbirth decisions.

Maternal mortality remains a critical public health issue with nearly 800 women dying daily from preventable causes related to pregnancy and childbirth.[75] The vast majority of these deaths occur in low-, lower-, middle-income countries, where access to quality maternal healthcare is limited. In the United States, where maternal mortality is on the rise, heart disease and stroke serve as predominant causes.[76] Due to systemic racism and implicit bias of practitioners, Black women face almost three times the risk of mortality compared to their White counterparts, with 69.9 deaths per 100,000 live births occurring.[77] Complications such as severe bleeding, infections, and high blood pressure during pregnancy account for most of these deaths, underscoring the importance of access to comprehensive prenatal, childbirth, and postpartum care.

Addressing maternal mortality requires a multifaceted approach that includes strengthening healthcare systems, enhancing maternal health education, and addressing social determinants of health that contribute to disparities. By ensuring that all women have access to high-quality maternal healthcare, the international community can make significant strides in reducing maternal mortality, ultimately achieving the goal of safe childbirth for every woman, everywhere.

Abortion, a term that sparks extensive debate and varying emotions, is a medical procedure to terminate a pregnancy. The WHO reports that each year, almost half of all pregnancies—121 million—are unintended; six out of ten unintended pregnancies and three out of ten of all pregnancies end in induced abortion.[78] There are primarily two methods: in-clinic abortion and the abortion pill, both recognized for their safety and commonality. The essence of abortion lies in the deliberate steps taken to end a pregnancy, distinct from spontaneous abortions or miscarriages which occur without medical intervention. The reasons women opt for abortion are as varied as the individuals themselves, ranging from birth timing and limiting family size to more pressing concerns such as maternal health, financial instability, domestic violence, or the aftermath of rape or incest. It's a decision underscored by the need for autonomy over one's body and future, reflecting the complex tapestry of personal and societal factors.

The methods employed for abortion have evolved, offering safe options that include medication and surgery. Mifepristone is safer to take than Viagra, Penicillin, or Tylenol.[79] Surgical abortions are significantly safer than other procedures such as plastic surgery. The safety of legal abortions stands in stark contrast to the dangers of illegal abortions, which pose significant risks to women's health, underscoring the necessity for legal, safe, and accessible abortion services.

Globally, abortion is a common reality, with approximately seventy-three million procedures performed annually, nearly half of which are conducted under unsafe conditions.[80] This statistic highlights the disparity in access to safe abortion care, particularly in developing regions where restrictive laws and limited access to healthcare exacerbate the risk to women's health and lives. They drastically reduce maternal mortality, reflecting a critical public health perspective that champions access to abortion as a cornerstone of women's healthcare.

The foundation of laws, especially those governing healthcare and reproductive rights, must be rooted in accurate and contemporary scientific understanding. Today's medical protocols calculate the commencement of pregnancy as the last day of a woman's last period. This is paradoxically two weeks before the maturation and ovulation of an egg from the ovary. This historical reliance on menstrual cycles as a measure of pregnancy onset assumed that women cannot accurately pinpoint ovulation or intercourse dates. This distorts the actual gestational age where at the time of conception women would technically be considered two weeks pregnant. Such misinterpretation becomes critically consequential in United States' jurisdictions where abortion laws restrict access as early as six weeks post-conception, effectively reducing the window to merely four weeks of actual pregnancy. Clarifying and unifying the definition of pregnancy onset is crucial in advocating for abortion rights, ensuring laws align with scientific reality, and respecting women's autonomy over their bodies. This accurate framing is essential for informed public discourse and for creating policies that genuinely reflect the principles of health, autonomy, and justice.

Let's explore how FemTech innovators are improving the experience of pregnant and birthing people.

## Eric Dy, PhD, Founder and CEO at Bloomlife

*Bloomlife is designed to streamline the flow of information between patients and practitioners, reducing the need for unnecessary visits while simultaneously improving clinical decision-making. Its wearable monitor tracks uterine contractions and maternal and fetal heart rates.*
*Episode 70 aired December 9, 2020.*

## What are some of the biggest misconceptions about labor?

One of the most significant misconceptions about normal labor and delivery is that it follows a strict, predictable pattern. In reality, labor and delivery can vary significantly from one woman to another. What's normal for one woman might not be for another. This variance is not just in terms of duration but also the intensity and progression of labor. Historically, medical benchmarks for labor progress, like the dilation of the cervix over time, were based on limited and homogenous data. These benchmarks don't always account for the wide range of normal variations in labor among different women.

Another misconception is the over-medicalization of the birth process. While medical interventions are crucial and lifesaving in many cases, there's a tendency to overly rely on them even in standard, low-risk deliveries. This can lead to unnecessary procedures like C-sections, which, although sometimes necessary, are significant surgeries with their own risks and implications.

More research in this field is crucial for several reasons. First, we need to better understand the physiological differences in labor and delivery among different women. This understanding can lead to more personalized approaches to childbirth, where interventions are used judiciously, and the natural process is respected whenever safe and possible.

Second, with the advancement of technology, we can collect and analyze real-time data from a diverse population of pregnant women. This can provide us with more accurate and comprehensive insights into the various ways that normal labor and delivery can present. It's not just about redefining norms but also about recognizing and accommodating the wide range of typical experiences in childbirth.

Last, more research can help us identify early indicators of potential complications, leading to timely interventions that can save lives and reduce the risk of long-term health issues for both mother and child. At Bloomlife, we're working toward gathering such data to contribute to this understanding and help shift the paradigm in maternal healthcare toward more personalized, data-driven care.

## Tell us about the Bloomlife Product.

At the heart of Bloomlife is our wearable device, a small, matchbox-sized sensor that attaches to a patch worn on the pregnant woman's belly. This sensor is designed to noninvasively track various physiological signals related to maternal and fetal health throughout pregnancy. It can monitor uterine contractions, fetal heart rate, and maternal health parameters. Unlike traditional monitoring systems that are often bulky, uncomfortable, and can only be used in a clinical setting, our device is portable and user-friendly, allowing continuous monitoring in the comfort of a woman's home.

The technology behind Bloomlife is quite innovative. We use electrodes to pick up the electrical activity generated by uterine muscles and the fetal heart, which are both muscles and each have unique electrical signals. This allows us to gather rich data, not just about the frequency of contractions but also about the coordination of uterine muscle activity, which can provide insights into different stages of labor.

Our goals with Bloomlife are multifold. First, we aim to empower expectant mothers with knowledge about their own health and the health of their babies. By providing them with real-time data and insights, we can help them feel more connected, prepared, engaged, and reassured in their pregnancy journey

Second, we're focused on collecting a large, longitudinal physiological dataset across a diverse population of pregnant women. With this data, we aim to advance the science of obstetrics by developing digital biomarkers that could predict complications like preterm birth. Our goal is to create a paradigm shift in delivering prenatal care, making it more proactive rather than reactive.

Last, we aim to improve access to prenatal care, especially for women in underserved communities who might have barriers to accessing regular healthcare services. By providing remote monitoring capabilities, we can bridge some of these gaps and ensure that all women, regardless of their location, socioeconomic status, or type of birth they choose, will receive the care they need during pregnancy.

## Gabriela Gerhart, Founder at Motherhood Center

*Motherhood Center provides comprehensive support to mothers during pregnancy and postpartum through education and in-home care services. Episode 15 aired June 1, 2020.*

## What are the different birthing options that women have today?

Today, women have several birthing options to choose from, each offering a unique experience. The choice depends on individual preferences, health considerations, and sometimes the circumstances of the pregnancy. Let's look at the main options.

Hospital Birth: This is the most common choice. Hospitals offer the highest level of medical resources and emergency care. Many hospitals now have birthing centers within them that offer a more home-like environment while still providing access to medical interventions if needed.

Birthing Centers: These are a middle ground between a home birth and a hospital birth. They provide a more natural, less clinical environment, and are typically run by midwives. Birthing centers are equipped for natural births and often have facilities like birthing pools.

Home Birth: For a home birth, a woman remains in the comfort of her home, supported by a midwife or a trained birth attendant. This option is chosen for its familiar, intimate setting, and for the control it gives the mother over her birthing environment. However, it's essential to have a plan for rapid transfer to a hospital in case of complications.

Water Birth: This can occur at home, in a birthing center, or in some hospitals. It involves laboring and sometimes giving birth in a warm pool of water. Proponents believe it's more relaxing, helps with pain, and eases the baby's transition to the outside world.

Each option has pros and cons, and the choice largely depends on the mother's health, pregnancy, and personal preferences. Women must discuss these options with their healthcare providers to understand what is best for their unique situation.

## How could hospitals improve the birthing experience for women?

Hospitals can significantly enhance the birthing experience for women by focusing on a few key areas.

Personalizing Care: Every woman's birthing experience is unique, and personalized care can make a big difference. This includes respecting individual birth plans, providing continuous support during labor, and ensuring that the woman's preferences and needs are prioritized.

Creating a Comfortable Environment: Hospitals can make labor and delivery rooms more comfortable and less clinical. This could involve softer lighting, music options, and the availability of various birthing aids like birthing balls and tubs for water births. A welcoming environment can help reduce stress and anxiety for the mother.

Encouraging Family Involvement: Allowing and encouraging the involvement of partners or family members during labor and delivery can provide emotional support and comfort to the birthing mother. Hospitals could facilitate this by having policies that support the presence of loved ones, as long as medical conditions permit.

Offering Pain Management Options: Providing a range of pain management options, from epidurals to natural methods like breathing techniques, hydrotherapy, or acupuncture, allows women to choose what works best for them.

Providing Postpartum Support: The birthing experience doesn't end with delivery. Offering robust postpartum support, including lactation consultants, mental health resources, and educational materials about newborn care, can significantly impact a new mother's well-being.

Staff Training: Regular training of hospital staff in empathy, communication, and the latest birthing practices can ensure that women receive the best possible care. Staff should be trained to listen to and respect the wishes of the birthing mother.

Ensuring Emergency Preparedness: While focusing on natural and comfortable birthing experiences, hospitals should also ensure swift and efficient responses to emergencies. This balance is crucial for the safety and trust of the mothers.

Ultimately, the goal should be to make the birth experience as positive, safe, and empowering as possible, honoring the preferences and dignity of each woman. By implementing these improvements, hospitals can create an environment where women feel supported, respected, and in control of their birthing experience. Unfortunately, this is not a current guarantee for most women, especially women of color.

## Kimberly Seals Allers, Founder at Irth

*Irth is an app born out of the necessity for improved Black maternal outcomes. "Irth," standing for "birth" but dropping the "B" for bias, challenges the bias experienced by Black women in health settings by allowing people to leave reviews of their experiences. Simultaneously, it informs the community about racism in healthcare and provides hospitals with feedback to acknowledge and address their weaknesses.*

*Episode 60 aired November 4, 2020.*

**What is the role of racism in Black women's maternal health?**

We know that racism affects Black women's maternal health through a convergence of data, research, and lived experiences that consistently point to disparities that cannot be explained by factors other than race. Several key indicators illuminate this issue.

Disparities Transcending Socioeconomic Status: Studies have repeatedly shown that Black women, regardless of their income, education level, or access to healthcare, are still at a higher risk for adverse maternal outcomes compared to their White counterparts. This suggests that factors beyond socioeconomic status, like the impact of systemic racism, play a critical role.

Consistent Patterns Across the Healthcare System: There is a pattern of Black women receiving lower quality care, being less listened to, and having their pain and symptoms underestimated or ignored across various healthcare settings. These patterns are indicative of implicit biases and racist attitudes within the healthcare system.

Historical Context: The historical mistreatment of Black women in the healthcare system, including unethical medical experimentation and lack of consent, has created a legacy of distrust and fear, which impacts how Black women engage with healthcare providers. This history is rooted in racism and continues to influence maternal health outcomes today.

Stress of Racial Discrimination: The chronic stress associated with racial discrimination has been linked to adverse health outcomes. This stress, often referred to as "weathering," can lead to conditions like hypertension, which are risk factors for complications during pregnancy and childbirth.

Comparative International Data: When we look at countries with similar economic status but different racial dynamics, we see that the maternal health disparities experienced by Black women in the US are not as prevalent. This suggests that the unique racial landscape in the US is a significant contributing factor.

To address this, we need a multifaceted approach that includes policy changes, education, and training to combat implicit biases in healthcare, and a commitment to listening to and valuing the experiences of Black women. Only by acknowledging and actively working to dismantle the systemic racism in our healthcare system can we begin to improve maternal health outcomes for Black women.

**What is the Irth app? How does it work? What have you found so far?**

The core concept of Irth is grounded in the belief that the experiences of Black and Brown women in healthcare settings need to be heard, validated, and addressed to bring about meaningful change.

Here's how Irth works.

Yelp-like Reviews: The app functions similarly to Yelp but focuses explicitly on maternity care. It allows mothers and birthing people to leave reviews of their experiences with doctors, hospitals, and other healthcare providers.

Specific Focus on Bias and Racism: Unlike general review platforms, Irth is designed to capture nuances and specifics about experiences of bias, racism, or discrimination. This can include incidents where patients felt their concerns were dismissed, where they experienced differential treatment, or where they faced overt racism.

Aggregating Data for Change: These personal stories and reviews are not just anecdotal. Irth aggregates them into actionable data. This data can be used to highlight patterns of discrimination, identify problem areas, and hold healthcare providers and institutions accountable.

Our findings from the data collected through Irth have been eye-opening and confirm the urgency of addressing racial bias in healthcare. Here is some of what we've found.

Consistent Patterns of Disparities: Many Black and Brown women report feeling unheard, dismissed, or outright disrespected in their maternal healthcare journeys. This is a pervasive issue, not isolated to certain regions or specific healthcare providers.

Impact of Implicit Bias: The reviews often reveal implicit biases in how healthcare providers interact with patients of color. This includes assumptions about their knowledge, lifestyle, or pain tolerance.

The Power of Shared Experiences: By sharing their stories, women are helping identify problematic practices and empowering each other. They're creating a community of support and knowledge that can guide others in making informed choices about their maternal care.

A Tool for Advocacy and Change: The aggregated data from Irth is a powerful tool for advocacy. It provides concrete evidence that can be used to push for policy changes, improved training for healthcare providers, and overall systemic reform.

Overall, the Irth app is more than just a review platform; it's a movement toward equitable maternal healthcare. It's about giving voice to those who have been marginalized and using that collective voice to drive real, lasting change in the healthcare system. We know every aspect of birthing needs innovation, down to the medical device we use for common procedures.

## Barry McCann, Founder and CEO at Nua Surgical

*Nua Surgical has designed the SteriCISION C-Section Retractor to improve C-section technology. This tool will allow physicians to have unobstructed visualization and improved access during a C-section, with the primary goal of enhancing the efficacy and safety of the surgery.*
*Episode 175 aired August 8, 2022.*

### What are the risks and complications that come along with cesareans?

Cesarean sections, while common and often necessary, come with a range of challenges and potential complications. One of the primary challenges is ensuring safe and adequate access to the uterus. This can be particularly difficult in cases of obesity or other complications that increase the thickness of the abdominal wall. The traditional tools and methods used in C-sections, such as manual retractors and hands-on assistance, can be limited in their effectiveness and can add physical strain to both the patient and the surgical team.

Another significant challenge is the risk of infection. Since a C-section is a major abdominal surgery, it involves incisions through the skin and uterus, which increases the risk of bacterial contamination. Infections can occur at the incision site or within the uterus and can lead to longer hospital stays, additional treatments, and, in some cases, more severe health issues.

Blood loss is also a concern during and after a C-section. While blood loss is expected in any surgical procedure, excessive bleeding can lead to complications and may require additional interventions such as blood transfusions.

Additionally, C-sections can have longer recovery times compared to vaginal births. The physical recovery from the surgery can impact a mother's ability to care for her newborn in the immediate postpartum period. This includes challenges with mobility, pain management, and potential difficulties with breastfeeding.

Last, there are potential long-term implications for both the mother and the child. For the mother, repeated C-sections can increase the risk of complications in future pregnancies. For the child, there's emerging research suggesting possible long-term health impacts associated with being born via C-section, though this area is still under study.

## Tell us about Nua Surgical.

The idea for Nua Surgical and our flagship product, the SteriCISION C-section Retractor, was born out of my experience with the BioInnovate Ireland program, where I had the opportunity to deeply immerse myself in the field of obstetrics and gynecology. During this program, we conducted extensive clinical observations in hospitals and identified various unmet needs in women's health. One of the most striking challenges we observed was in cesarean section (C-section) surgeries.

During C-section procedures, we noticed that the existing surgical tools and methods were often inadequate, especially in handling the increased complexity of surgeries due to factors like obesity. We saw that surgeons frequently relied on manual methods for retracting the surgical site, which not only increased the physical strain on the medical staff but also posed higher risks of complications like infections and excessive bleeding for the patients.

This observation led us to develop the SteriCISION C-section Retractor, a medical device specifically designed for C-sections. Our device is a single-use, disposable retractor that provides enhanced ergonomics and functionality during the surgery. It is designed to improve access and visualization of the uterus, thereby making the procedure safer and more efficient.

The key features of our device include adjustable paddles with a soft touch, which are gentle on the patient's body, reducing the risk of tissue trauma. The device's design allows for easy deployment, providing optimal retraction with minimal need for manual assistance. This improves the surgical process and reduces the risk of infection by minimizing the number of hands and tools needed at the surgical site. We know it's not a simple road to having a baby; let us make the final stretch of the process less risky.

## Lina Chan, Founder and CEO at Parla

*Parla is an expert-led community designed to support women through various health challenges, with a particular focus on the mental and emotional aspects of women's health, including the journey through miscarriage. Episode 135 aired October 5, 2021.*

**How does miscarriage affect women's mental health?**

Miscarriage is a highly common yet underdiscussed experience, affecting one in four pregnancies. This significant occurrence is the leading complication in pregnancies, yet the societal and health systems' support for women undergoing this trauma is insufficient. The pervasive silence around miscarriage, coupled with the advice often given to women not to disclose their pregnancies until after the first trimester, exacerbates the isolation and lack of support women feel during this time. This practice stems from the high incidence of miscarriage within the first twelve weeks, yet it also strips women of their natural support systems when they need them most.

The impact of miscarriage on women's mental health is profound, with 70 percent of women who experience pregnancy loss showing symptoms of PTSD. This statistic underscores the urgent need for healthcare systems to offer more than just physical care and integrate mental health support as a standard part of miscarriage care. Currently, the healthcare system's approach to miscarriage is starkly inadequate, with women expected to endure multiple losses before receiving in-depth medical investigation or support in many cases. This gap in care reflects a broader issue within women's health, where mental and emotional well-being is often overlooked.

Despite the prevalence and significant impact of miscarriage, the conversation around it remains muted, contributing to the stigma and isolation women face. The societal impulse to keep early pregnancy and its potential loss a secret only compounds the emotional distress, leaving women to navigate their grief without the necessary support. This silence around miscarriage and the lack of comprehensive care reflect critical areas of women's health that demand attention, advocacy, and innovation to ensure that women and families receive the holistic support they need during one of life's most challenging moments.

### What is Parla? Why did you start it?

Parla provides curated programs that combine the expertise of clinical psychologists, nutritionists, and fertility nurses to offer a holistic approach to care after miscarriage. Experts craft our content, which includes meditations, journaling prompts, and access to peer support, all aimed at empowering women to navigate their emotions and experiences more healthily.

The emotional turmoil following a miscarriage is profound, often leading to symptoms akin to PTSD. Recognizing this, Parla's miscarriage support program is centered around mental health, offering resources and support that address the grief, isolation, and emotional pain that accompany pregnancy loss. By integrating these elements into our platform, we aim to break the silence around miscarriage, providing women with the understanding and support they need during such a vulnerable time.

I was motivated to start Parla following my personal struggles with pregnancy loss and the realization of the glaring gaps in support and information available to women undergoing similar experiences. The journey left me deeply aware of the impact of mental health on physical health and the need for a more integrated, compassionate approach to women's healthcare. Parla embodies this mission, striving to create a space where women can find comprehensive support, expertise, and community, all tailored to their unique health and emotional needs. There are many times and experiences during pregnancy when women and girls need extra emotional support.

## Roopan Gill, MD, MPH FRCSC, Cofounder and CEO at Vitala Global

*Vitala Global is addressing the global need for safe and accessible abortion care, particularly in low- and middle-income countries.*
*Episode 65 aired November 23, 2020.*

### What is Vitala Global and why did you start it?

Vitala Global was born out of a deep-seated passion for addressing the needs of women and girls in accessing sexual and reproductive health services, particularly in areas that are often stigmatized like abortion and contraception. As an obstetrician-gynecologist specializing in family planning, my experiences in Canada and in various other global health contexts have consistently highlighted the immense gaps and challenges in this sector.

Our mission is to codesign digital solutions that empower individuals, especially in challenging contexts, to manage their own abortions and family-planning needs. This need became even more apparent during my time with Médecins Sans Frontières and at the WHO, where I witnessed firsthand the consequences of inadequate access to safe abortion and family-planning services.

Vitala Global stands at the intersection of activism, academia, and technology, aiming to bridge gaps and normalize conversations around abortion and miscarriage. Our work is a testament to the fact that comprehensive abortion care is a critical aspect of women's health that requires innovative, empathetic, and multidisciplinary approaches. We are committed to ensuring that women have the support and resources they need to make informed decisions about their reproductive health, no matter where they are.

## What is a self-administered abortion?

A self-administered abortion, also known as a self-managed abortion, involves a pregnant person safely terminating their pregnancy using medication, specifically mifepristone and misoprostol, or misoprostol alone, without the direct supervision of a healthcare provider. This method is recognized as safe and effective by the World Health Organization, particularly within the first ten weeks of pregnancy.

In a self-managed abortion, the individual assesses their eligibility for the medication, taking into consideration factors like the duration of pregnancy and their overall health. They then self-administer the medication, usually at home or in a comfortable environment of their choosing. It's important that during this process, they have access to accurate information and understand the proper use of the medication, the expected symptoms, and how to identify any complications.

The emphasis on self-managed abortion is increasingly significant, especially in areas with restricted access to abortion services or where legal barriers exist. It empowers individuals to take control of their reproductive health, especially when supported by reliable information and, if needed, access to follow-up medical care. The key to safe self-managed abortion is ensuring the availability of accurate information and support, which can come from various sources including digital platforms, hotlines, and community health workers.

For example, in Latin America, the state of abortion varies significantly across countries, reflecting a mosaic of laws and cultural attitudes. Many countries have restrictive abortion laws, permitting abortion only in limited circumstances, such as to save the woman's life or in cases of rape. These restrictions often drive women toward unsafe methods, posing significant health risks.

### Why is emotional support after an abortion so critical?

Emotional support after an abortion is critical because the experience of abortion, irrespective of the circumstances, can be emotionally complex. Women may experience a range of feelings from relief to sadness, or even guilt, influenced by personal beliefs, societal attitudes, and the stigma that often surrounds abortion. Quality emotional support helps cope with these feelings, ensuring that women feel understood, respected, and not isolated in their experience. This support is not just about managing immediate emotional responses, but also about empowering women, reaffirming their autonomy, and aiding them in making informed decisions about their reproductive health in the future. It's about acknowledging and addressing the whole spectrum of needs—physical, emotional, and psychological—that contribute to a woman's well-being post-abortion.

* * *

The pregnancy chapter encapsulates the intricate and profound journey of gestation, marked by a nuanced understanding of the physiological, emotional, and societal shifts accompanying this transformative period. It delves into the stages of fetal development across three trimesters, each critical for the distinct milestones from organ formation to preparing for birth, with a clear exposition on the common yet seldom discussed phenomena such as miscarriages and the varying complications that can arise, emphasizing the stark disparities in maternal health outcomes across different demographics. The narrative also explores the evolution of childbirth practices, from ancient reliance on midwives to the modern medicalized approach, highlighting ongoing debates about the optimal balance between natural and assisted birthing methods. This discussion extends into the repercussions of cesarean sections and the role of epidurals in labor, reflecting broader trends and concerns within maternal healthcare. Notably, the chapter does not shy away from addressing systemic issues, such as racial disparities and the need for comprehensive prenatal and postpartum care, advocating for a more equitable and empathetic healthcare framework that supports all women through the challenges and triumphs of pregnancy.

# Chapter 8
# Breastfeeding

**ELIZA, A DEDICATED KINDERGARTEN TEACHER** passionate about her profession, eagerly anticipated the birth of her first child. She adored her job, nurturing young minds with the same care she planned to give her own child. However, as her due date approached, Eliza faced a harsh reality that clouded her excitement. Aware of the demanding nature of her job and the lack of private spaces and breaks to pump breast milk, she realized that breastfeeding would not be feasible. It struck her profoundly that her female-dominated field, seemingly attuned to the needs of children, lacked the necessary accommodations for new mothers to balance their professional responsibilities with the natural act of breastfeeding.

Eliza's disillusionment grew as she delved into the policies—or the lack thereof—that would support her postpartum. The absence of structured support for breastfeeding in her workplace was a bitter pill to swallow, highlighting a significant oversight in a sector filled with women, many of whom were mothers themselves. She was dismayed that despite the known benefits of breastfeeding, there were no provisions to enable her to provide her baby with the best start in life. This revelation affected her personal planning and sparked a desire in Eliza to advocate for change. She began campaigning for better maternity accommodations and determined that no other woman in her field should have to forgo the invaluable breastfeeding experience due to workplace constraints.

Breastfeeding stands as the pinnacle of infant nutrition, offering many health benefits beyond mere sustenance. Despite its critical role, current statistics reveal that only one in four infants is exclusively breastfed by the six-month mark, a figure starkly below global health recommendations.[81] This shortfall not only compromises child and maternal health but also imposes an economic burden exceeding $3 billion annually in medical costs within the United States alone.[82]

Global health authorities, including WHO and UNICEF, advocate for exclusive breastfeeding during the initial six months of an infant's life, followed by continued breastfeeding complemented with appropriate foods for up to two years or beyond. This recommendation is rooted in extensive research underscoring the unparalleled benefits of breast milk in fostering infant health and development.

Breastfeeding is a complex biological process driven by hormonal signals, primarily prolactin and oxytocin. These hormones facilitate milk production and release, adapting to the infant's needs through a sophisticated feedback mechanism related to the degree of breast emptiness or fullness with the emptier breast producing milk faster than the fuller one. Milk production is also responsive to maternal states of well-being, with stress and fatigue adversely impacting supply; relaxation is key for successful lactation.[83] Milk synthesis remains surprisingly constant at approximately 800mL/d and is finely tuned to demand, with the composition of breast milk evolving to meet the nutritional requirements of the growing infant.[84] For example, early milk or colostrum has lower concentrations of fat than mature milk but higher concentrations of protein and minerals.

The concept of wet nurses, lactating women who nurse children other than their own, has a profound historical footprint. Once a prevalent practice, wet nursing offered a solution for mothers unable to breastfeed for various reasons. However, the advent of infant formula and changing societal norms have rendered this practice nearly obsolete, although it raises questions about contemporary alternatives in the face of breastfeeding challenges.

Breastfeeding's history is as diverse as it is long, reflecting societal values, technological advancements, and economic conditions. The emergence of infant formula in the nineteenth century marked a significant turning point, influencing breastfeeding rates and practices. Despite these shifts, the twentieth century witnessed a resurgence in breastfeeding advocacy, highlighting its health benefits and importance.

Today, breastfeeding faces numerous challenges, from societal and cultural stigmas to aggressive marketing of breast milk substitutes. These obstacles are compounded by a lack of support in healthcare settings and workplaces, alongside pervasive myths and misconceptions about breastfeeding.

Racial and socioeconomic disparities in breastfeeding rates are significant, with Black infants in the United States less likely to be breastfed compared to their counterparts (77 percent versus the national average of 83 percent).[85,86]These disparities are not merely a matter of personal choice but are deeply rooted in centuries of oppressive laws, historical injustices, systemic barriers, and targeted marketing practices that have systematically undermined breastfeeding among marginalized communities. In 1981, the US didn't sign onto the World Health Organization's International Code of Marketing Breastmilk Substitutes, which unconsciously allowed unrestricted advertisements encouraging Black mothers to formula-feed initially even when they couldn't afford it in the long term. This inequality continues today: Black newborns are nine times more likely to get formula in hospitals compared with White babies.[87]

Rates of breastfeeding differ around the globe, with initiation almost universal in African, Asian, and some South American regions. In European countries, we see this variation more starkly, with just 81 percent of mothers starting to breastfeed in the UK compared to almost all mothers in Nordic regions initiating breastfeeding and three-quarters continuing until six months postpartum.[88] Education level, age, profession, and ethnic background all influence the rates of breastfeeding.

A concerted effort is needed to bridge the gap in breastfeeding rates and ensure all infants benefit from the optimal nutrition it provides. This involves comprehensive support for breastfeeding mothers, inclusive policies that accommodate breastfeeding in public and workplaces, and targeted initiatives to counteract the misinformation and stigma surrounding breastfeeding.

Breastfeeding is critical to maternal and child health, offering a foundation for lifelong health benefits. However, realizing its full potential requires overcoming historical legacies, cultural barriers, and contemporary challenges through informed policies, community support, and public health initiatives. As we move forward, it is imperative to embrace breastfeeding not only as a biological necessity but as a societal responsibility, ensuring that every child has the best start in life. FemTech companies are making significant strides with innovative products to elevate the breastfeeding experience.

## Etta Watts-Russell, Founder and CEO at Lactamo

*Lactamo is a developer of breast massage equipment designed to promote healthy breastfeeding. The company's product uses a combination of temperature, movement, and compression to help with common breast-feeding problems including oversupply, undersupply, blocked ducts, and engorgement. Episode 136 aired October 5, 2021.*

### What health challenges do breastfeeding women face?

Breastfeeding, though a natural process, can be fraught with several common yet challenging conditions that affect a vast majority of nursing mothers, with statistics indicating that up to 92 percent encounter difficulties. These challenges not only include physical discomforts but also serious health conditions that can significantly impact the breastfeeding experience.

Pain during breastfeeding can arise from various sources, including the baby's latch, nipple damage, or infections. Mothers must seek guidance from lactation consultants to ensure proper technique and promptly address any underlying issues.

Blocked ducts occur when milk flow through one of the many milk ducts in the breast is obstructed. This can lead to discomfort and swelling in the affected area. Blocked ducts are often caused by insufficient breast emptying, tight clothing, or infrequent feedings. Solutions include frequent breastfeeding, applying warm compresses, and gentle massage toward the nipple to encourage milk flow.

Engorgement is the painful overfilling of the breasts with milk, often accompanied by swelling and tenderness. It usually occurs when the milk supply adjusts to the baby's needs, especially in the early days of breast-feeding. Managing engorgement involves regular feeding, expressing milk to comfort, and using cold packs to reduce swelling.

Mastitis is a painful infection of the breast tissue that occurs in about 20 percent of breastfeeding women. It can result from unresolved blocked ducts, leading to inflammation and infection. Symptoms include fever, flu-like symptoms, and red, tender areas on the breast. Mastitis requires prompt medical attention, and treatment typically involves antibiotics, continued breastfeeding or milk expression, and warm compresses to alleviate discomfort.

The emotional toll of dealing with these conditions, on top of societal pressures to breastfeed successfully, adds a significant psychological burden on nursing mothers. Current solutions emphasize the importance of preventive measures, such as proper breastfeeding techniques and regular breast care, and the need for accessible, professional support from lactation consultants and healthcare providers. They underscore the necessity for comprehensive care approaches that address breastfeeding mothers' physical and emotional well-being.

## What is Lactamo?

Lactamo is a unique, therapeutic ball designed specifically for breastfeeding mothers facing common nursing challenges. I created Lactamo from personal experience and the realization that while breastfeeding is a natural process, it doesn't come naturally to all mothers. Up to 92 percent of nursing mothers encounter issues such as blocked ducts, engorgement, pain, over or undersupply of milk, and mastitis. These challenges can make breastfeeding a daunting task, and I wanted to provide a solution that empowers mothers to overcome these hurdles and have a more positive breastfeeding journey.

Lactamo works on the principle of temperature, movement, and compression. It's a soft, spherical tool made from medical-grade silicone, filled with a special gel that can be warmed or cooled according to the mother's needs. Applying Lactamo with gentle massage movements toward the nipple helps to stimulate milk flow, relieve blockages, reduce pain and swelling, and can even improve milk quality. The design is based on extensive research and developed in collaboration with lactation consultants to ensure it effectively addresses the myriad of breastfeeding issues. It's a simple, reusable, and affordable solution to make breastfeeding more manageable and less stressful for mothers. Because being able to express milk is the first major hurdle breastfeeders face. The next stress is typically knowing how much milk their baby consumes.

## Rosanne Longmore, Cofounder and CEO at Coroflo

*Coroflo created Coro, the world's first accurate breastfeeding monitor. It is a nipple shield that accurately measures the flow of breast milk. This data is connected to an app that records feed duration, time, and volume. Episode 227 aired January 31, 2024.*

### Why would it be helpful to quantify breast milk?

Quantifying breast milk is fundamentally important for several reasons. First, it provides crucial reassurance to mothers. Many women who choose to breastfeed face anxiety and uncertainty about whether their baby is receiving enough milk. This uncertainty is one of the top reasons why women stop breastfeeding earlier than they desire. By quantifying breast milk, mothers can have real-time data on the volume of milk their baby is consuming, which can alleviate concerns about underfeeding or overfeeding.

Additionally, quantifying breast milk has significant implications for medical and academic research. Until now, we've been operating in a vacuum of information regarding breast milk production and consumption. With accurate measurement, researchers can study variables that affect breast milk supply, such as maternal diet, health conditions, medication, and even the psychological factors involved in breastfeeding. This information is crucial for understanding and improving breastfeeding practices globally.

Furthermore, quantifying breast milk can help develop better healthcare strategies and policies to support breastfeeding mothers. It allows us to create more tailored and effective lactation support programs and address specific challenges that women face during breastfeeding. In essence, the ability to quantify breast milk empowers women with knowledge and choice, leading to more informed and confident decisions about their breastfeeding journey.

### How does Coroflo product work?

Coroflo is an innovative breakthrough in breastfeeding technology. It's the world's first accurate breastfeeding monitor, designed to empower mothers by providing real-time data on how much breast milk their baby consumes. The way Coroflo works is quite simple yet technologically advanced.

At its core, Coroflo features a standard silicone nipple shield, a familiar item to many breastfeeding mothers. This shield is equipped with our groundbreaking micro-flow sensor technology. When a mother breastfeeds her baby using the Coroflo shield, the sensor accurately measures the milk the baby consumes. This data is then transmitted in real-time to an accompanying app on the mother's phone.

What sets Coroflo apart is its precision and ease of use. The shield is ultra-thin and comfortable, ensuring the natural breastfeeding experience is preserved. The mother simply needs to wear the shield, and as she feeds her baby, she can observe the volume of milk consumed on the app. This real-time feedback is incredibly empowering, giving mothers assurance and confidence in their breastfeeding journey.

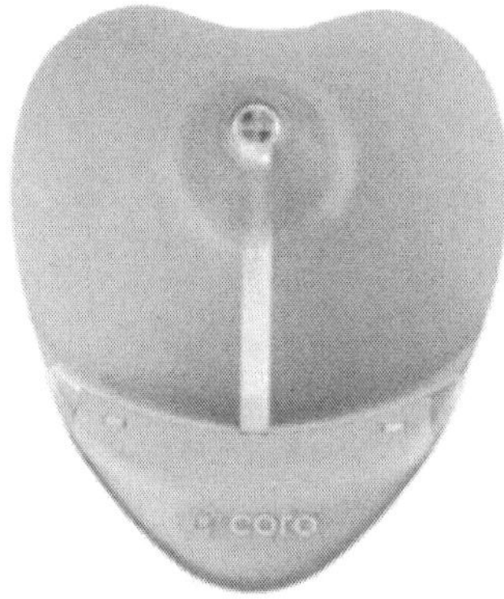


*Figure 12. Coroflo's proprietary nipple shield measures the amount of breast milk a baby drinks.*

After use, the shield can be easily washed and air-dried. It's designed for convenience and hygiene, ensuring mothers can use it seamlessly in daily routines.

Furthermore, Coroflo's technology goes beyond just assisting individual mothers. The data collected has immense potential for academic and medical research, enabling a deeper understanding of breastfeeding patterns, milk supply variables, and overall infant health. Scientists are growing interested in studying breast milk and have brought some of their laboratory technology mainstream to consumers.

## Berkley Luck, PhD, and Pedro Silva, Cofounders at Milkify

*Milkify is a provider of breast milk freeze-drying services intended to help moms overcome barriers to breast milk storage and transportation at*

*home and at work. The company offers breast milk powder that can be stored for years without refrigeration and can be used by mixing with warm purified water, just like powdered formula.*
*Episode 71 aired December 14, 2020.*

## What is Milkify, and what is the process of freeze-drying breast milk?

The inception of Milkify was rooted in a simple observation and a scientific background. While working on my research, which involved the infant gut microbiome and the preservation of bacteria through freeze-drying, I saw a colleague struggling with storing her pumped breast milk. It struck me that the same technology we use in the lab could revolutionize how breast milk is stored and used by breastfeeding mothers.

Milkify is essentially a service that transforms frozen breast milk into a shelf-stable powder through lyophilization, or freeze-drying. This process removes the water from the breast milk, leaving behind a dry powder that retains fresh breast milk's nutritional and immunological benefits. The powder can be stored for years without refrigeration and reconstituted with water.

Freeze-drying breast milk with Milkify is designed to be straightforward and stress-free for mothers. It starts with them sending us their frozen breast milk using our specially designed shipping kits, which ensure the milk stays frozen in transit. Once we receive the milk, it undergoes our proprietary freeze-drying process.

The milk is first deeply frozen during freeze-drying and then placed under a vacuum. This lets the ice sublimate directly into vapor, skipping the liquid phase. We apply gentle heat to facilitate this process, preserving the milk's delicate proteins, antibodies, and nutrients.

After freeze-drying, the milk is sealed in a moisture and oxygen-proof packaging to maintain its integrity. We then ship the powdered milk back to the mothers, to rehydrate it with sterilized water. This entire freeze-drying process is carried out in our facilities, adhering to strict quality control and safety standards to ensure the best possible product.

## What are the current challenges women face when storing breast milk?

Women currently store their breast milk primarily through refrigeration or freezing. However, these methods come with their own set of challenges and limitations. Freezing breast milk, while extending its shelf life, can lead to degradation of essential nutrients over time. Additionally, frozen breast milk requires careful thawing and can only be stored for a limited period before its quality diminishes. This process can be inconvenient for women, especially those who need to travel, work, or are unable to breastfeed directly due to various circumstances.

The risks of freezing breast milk include potential nutrient loss and the need for meticulous management to prevent bacterial contamination during thawing. Frozen milk must be used within a certain timeframe, typically six months to a year, to ensure its safety and nutritional value. This constraint demands careful planning and can contribute to stress for breastfeeding mothers trying to manage their milk supply.

Liquid or frozen breast milk's inconvenience stems from its storage requirements, the need for constant refrigeration, and the logistic challenges of transporting and thawing it. The fear of power outages or improper storage leading to spoiled milk is a constant concern, which can result in wasted milk and resources. For working mothers or those on the go, managing a supply of liquid breast milk can be cumbersome, limiting their mobility and adding to the complexities of motherhood. We know that working mothers who are breastfeeding need as many resources and support as possible.

## Abbey Donnell, Founder and CEO at Work & Mother

*Work & Mother addresses balancing work and motherhood by providing full-service mothers' rooms for commercial office buildings. These rooms offer mothers private and comfortable areas to pump, ensuring companies can meet the Fair Labor Standards Act (FLSA) Regulations and support mothers transitioning back to work without compromising their breastfeeding goals. Episode 20 aired June 17, 2020.*

### What challenges do women face when trying to pump at work?

Women face numerous challenges when trying to breast pump at work, reflecting a widespread issue across various workplace environments. Despite some companies being ostensibly family-friendly, many still lack adequate facilities for breastfeeding mothers, leading to situations where women resort to pumping in bathrooms, closets, or even cars due to the absence of a private, comfortable space. This problem is not confined to specific industries and affects women in predominantly female workplaces and male-dominated fields, like oil and gas companies.

The open office floor plan prevalent in modern workspaces exacerbates these challenges, offering no privacy for pumping. Employers often react by converting existing spaces like offices or closets into makeshift lactation rooms, but these solutions are typically inadequate, highlighting the necessity for dedicated, purpose-built facilities. The lack of proper lactation spaces not only poses logistic hurdles but also impacts mothers' emotional well-being and productivity, as they navigate the complexities of balancing work and breastfeeding.

Statistically, the drop-off rate in breastfeeding upon returning to work is significant. This stark decline is attributed to the challenges of pumping at work, including the absence of supportive facilities and the logistic nightmare of transporting and storing breast milk. The situation is further complicated by a baby's developmental milestones, such as growth spurts and sleep regressions, which can disrupt breastfeeding routines and exacerbate the difficulties faced by working mothers.

Moreover, the legal landscape around breastfeeding at work is evolving, with increasing recognition of the need for better support and facilities. However, progress is uneven and often depends on the presence of women in decision-making roles within companies and government. This underscores the importance of advocacy and policy development to create a more supportive environment for breastfeeding mothers in the workplace.

**What is Work & Mother? How are you helping businesses be compliant?**

Work & Mother is a comprehensive solution designed to address the challenges faced by breastfeeding mothers returning to the workforce. It offers fully equipped lactation facilities that cater to the needs of working moms, enabling them to pump during the workday without the logistic hassles commonly associated with this process. Each facility has hospital-grade pumps, cleaning supplies, and personal storage, creating a seamless and efficient experience for mothers.

This service is particularly beneficial for employers striving to comply with federal requirements to provide appropriate lactation spaces. By partnering with Work & Mother, businesses can easily meet these legal obligations without the need to retrofit their own spaces or create temporary solutions that may fall short of their employees' needs. Work & Mother's facilities ensure privacy, security, and convenience, offering a dedicated space that effectively supports breastfeeding employees.

Work & Mother presents a practical and cost-effective solution for office buildings and small businesses. Many small businesses may lack the resources or space to set up their own lactation rooms. By integrating Work & Mother facilities into their buildings, property managers can offer a valuable amenity that attracts and retains tenants, particularly those businesses committed to supporting their employees' work-life balance. This approach enhances the building's appeal and helps small businesses provide a supportive environment for working mothers, ultimately contributing to employee satisfaction and retention. Many employers are becoming serious about supporting their breastfeeding employees, including those who travel.

## Kate Torgersen, Founder and CEO at Milk Stork

*Milk Stork provides breast milk shipping services to help moms maintain their commitment to breastfeeding, especially for women who travel for work. They offer domestic and international delivery options, enabling mothers to focus on work and care for their babies conveniently.*
*Episode 26 aired July 8, 2020.*

### Why should employers be supporting their breastfeeding employees?

Women working while breastfeeding face numerous challenges, including the logistic difficulties of pumping at work, maintaining milk supply, and balancing professional responsibilities with the demands of breastfeeding. These challenges are further exacerbated by the lack of supportive workplace policies, such as inadequate lactation spaces and inflexible work schedules, making it difficult for women to continue breastfeeding upon returning to work.

Employers should support breastfeeding mothers because it benefits employees and the organization. Supporting breastfeeding can lower healthcare costs, reduce absenteeism, increase employee retention, and improve morale and job satisfaction among working mothers. By providing lactation support, employers demonstrate a commitment to family-friendly policies, which can enhance their reputation and attractiveness.

The benefits of supporting breastfeeding mothers in the workplace include healthier babies and mothers, leading to lower healthcare costs and fewer sick days taken to care for ill children. Breastfeeding support can also increase employee loyalty and retention, as women are more likely to return to work and remain with an employer that accommodates their breastfeeding needs. Additionally, supporting breastfeeding contributes to a positive company culture and can improve overall employee satisfaction and productivity.

The consequences of not supporting breastfeeding mothers include higher healthcare costs due to increased infant illness, lower employee morale and job satisfaction, and potential legal ramifications from failing to comply with laws that protect breastfeeding rights. Lack of support can lead to decreased breastfeeding rates, which impacts the health and well-being of both mothers and their children. Furthermore, companies may face challenges in retaining talented female employees who may seek more supportive work environments.

**What is Milk Stork?**

Milk Stork is the first and leading breast milk shipping service, designed to support breastfeeding mothers who need to travel for work or other reasons. I started it out of personal necessity, after experiencing the logistic nightmare of trying to maintain my milk supply for my twins while on a business trip. I realized there was a significant gap in support for working breastfeeding mothers. The service enables moms to ship or carry their expressed milk back to their babies, ensuring they can continue breastfeeding without interruption, regardless of location or schedule.

Women have been incredibly vocal about Milk Stork's transformative impact on their breastfeeding journeys and careers. They often describe the service as a game-changer, allowing them to return to work, travel as needed, and achieve their breastfeeding goals without compromise. The relief and gratitude expressed by these mothers underscore the critical need for such support in balancing career ambitions with maternal responsibilities.

Employers, too, have recognized the value of Milk Stork, not just as a benefit for their breastfeeding employees but as a strategic investment in their workforce. By offering Milk Stork as part of their benefits package, companies send a powerful message about their commitment to support families and gender equality in the workplace. This has become essential to attracting and retaining top female talent, enhancing employee satisfaction, and promoting a family-friendly corporate culture. The employer business model has proven to be an excellent revenue stream for women's health companies like Milk Stork because it aligns businesses' interests with their employees' well-being, creating a win-win scenario. It's not just about providing a service; it's about fostering an inclusive workplace where women feel valued and supported in all aspects of their lives, including motherhood.

* * *

The chapter on breastfeeding encapsulates the myriad challenges and profound benefits associated with this natural yet complex act of nurturing. Despite its well-documented health advantages for both mother and child, breastfeeding rates remain suboptimal due to a confluence of social, cultural, and logistic barriers. The chapter addresses these issues, advocating for enhanced societal and employer support, including adequate maternity leave, flexible working conditions, and accessible lactation spaces. Moreover, it underscores the importance of dispelling myths and providing education about breastfeeding's benefits, positioning it not just as a personal choice but a public health imperative. By fostering a supportive environment, we can ensure that breastfeeding is a feasible, embraced practice that contributes to healthier generations and a more understanding society.

# Chapter 9
# Pelvic Floor

**MARGARET, A SPIRITED WOMAN** with a profound love for gardening, had recently embraced the serene pace of countryside retirement, a stark contrast to her bustling life as a mother of three. The gardens she tended were not just plots of land, but sanctuaries where she found peace and purpose. However, decades of struggling with a weak pelvic floor after childbirth had cast a shadow over her golden years. Despite faithfully following the age-old advice of performing Kegels, promised to remedy her condition, Margaret found her situation worsening with age. Activities that once brought her joy, like tending to her beloved garden, were marred by the fear of urinary leakage. This issue intensified her isolation and impacted her active lifestyle dramatically.

The real test of her resolve came in social settings; dinner parties with friends and family became sources of anxiety rather than joy when she could not control flatulence. The embarrassment was palpable, adding a layer of distress to her interactions. Eventually, Margaret resorted to buying adult diapers, a decision that, while practical, deeply wounded her pride and intensified her feelings of shame. Her struggle with incontinence, once a private battle, was now a barrier that limited her engagement in her cherished activities and social life. Faced with these challenges, Margaret realized that her quality of life hinged on seeking more effective medical solutions beyond the traditional advice she had been given. This realization propelled her to consult specialists who could offer new treatments and technologies, sparking hope that she could regain control and fully embrace the joys of her retirement without restraint.

The pelvic floor is pivotal in the human body's structural integrity and functional prowess. Nestled within the pelvis, the pelvic floor muscles act as a supportive sling for the pelvic organs, including the bladder, the bowels, and, in females, the uterus. These muscles stretch from the pubic bone at the front to the coccyx or tailbone at the back, forming the group's foundation, commonly called the core. Beyond their supportive role, the pelvic floor muscles are integral to bladder and bowel control, sexual function, and, in females, supporting the baby during pregnancy and then facilitating childbirth.

Pelvic floor disorders (PFDs) can manifest due to weakened, overstretched, or overly tight pelvic floor muscles. Factors contributing to such conditions include pregnancy, childbirth, obesity, chronic constipation, and surgeries like prostatectomy. Symptoms of PFDs range from incontinence and pelvic organ prolapse to sexual dysfunction and chronic pelvic pain, affecting an individual's quality of life profoundly.

The prevalence of PFDs among women is both startling and sobering, with one in three women expected to experience a PFD in her lifetime.[89] These disorders, which include urinary incontinence, pelvic organ prolapse, and other lower urinary tract symptoms, affect at least 25 percent of women in the United States and as high as 47 percent in countries like Japan.[90] The economic impact of managing and treating these conditions is substantial, with the total annual cost of urinary incontinence management alone reaching €69.1 billion in Europe in 2023, projected to increase by 25 percent in 2030 to €86.7 billion.[91] Furthermore, the cost associated with pelvic organ prolapse surgery in the US alone has surged to over $1.5 billion annually, highlighting a growing need for both outpatient and inpatient care.[92] Despite their high prevalence and significant economic burden, PFDs often remain undiagnosed or undertreated, compounded by patient embarrassment and a lack of awareness, ultimately taking a toll on the quality of life, social engagement, and emotional well-being of those affected.

The historical use of mesh and dilators for treating PFDs like pelvic organ prolapse (POP) and stress urinary incontinence (SUI) has a complex and often troubling legacy. Initially, mesh was introduced in the 1950s for abdominal hernias, but by the 1990s, it found a new application in gynecology for repairing POP and SUI. This innovation was initially embraced due to its perceived benefits over traditional tissue repair methods. However, the enthusiasm waned as the adverse effects became apparent, leading to significant discomfort, pain, and harm to many women. The FDA's increasing concern over these complications prompted regulatory actions, culminating in reclassifying transvaginal mesh for POP repair as a high-risk device in 2016 and the eventual ban of most transvaginal mesh products in 2019. The aftermath has seen legal battles and billions in compensation for the affected women.

Similarly, vaginal dilators, first introduced in 1938, have been recommended for various conditions, including post-radiation therapy and congenital malformations. Despite their potential benefits, the use of dilators has been marred by reports of pain, discomfort, and psychological distress, contributing to low adherence rates among women. This lack of compliance underscores the complex interplay between the physical and emotional aspects of PFD treatment.

These historical solutions to PFDs, mesh, and dilators, though innovative at their inception, have often resulted in more harm than good, underscoring an urgent need for innovation in this field. The journey from widespread adoption to controversy and legal action highlights the importance of safety, efficacy, and patient well-being in developing medical treatments for PFDs.

Enter the pelvic floor therapist—a specialized physiotherapist equipped with the knowledge and skills to diagnose and treat PFDs. Through a combination of techniques such as manual therapy, biofeedback, electrical stimulation, and targeted exercises, pelvic floor therapists tailor rehabilitation programs to address each patient's unique needs.

Pelvic floor muscle training (PFMT), known as Kegel exercises, is the cornerstone of pelvic floor strengthening. Correctly identifying and engaging these muscles is the first step, followed by a regimen of exercises designed to improve muscle tone, endurance, and control. Regular, consistent practice of PFMT can significantly enhance bladder and bowel function, sexual health, and overall pelvic stability.

Advancements in research and treatment methodologies continue to enhance our understanding of pelvic floor health. Studies exploring the efficacy of various rehabilitation techniques, the impact of lifestyle changes, and the development of innovative therapeutic tools all promise to expand the horizons of PFD management.

Though often overlooked, the pelvic floor is a vital component of our body's core stability and functional integrity. Recognizing its importance, addressing injuries and dysfunctions with informed care, and embracing preventive measures can improve health outcomes and quality of life. As awareness grows and innovative FemTech treatment approaches evolve, the future of pelvic floor health looks promising, offering hope and relief to millions affected by PFDs worldwide.

## Rachel Bartholomew, Founder and CEO at Hyivy

*Hyivy is a pelvic rehabilitation company offering devices that track data for customers with pelvic diseases, aiding in their recovery.*
*Episode 67 aired November 30, 2020.*

### What is the female pelvic floor, and what role does it play in women's health?

It's a network of muscles, ligaments, and tissues that stretch like a hammock from the pubic bone to the tailbone, supporting the uterus, bladder, and rectum. Its health is crucial for several reasons.

First, a strong and functional pelvic floor is essential for bladder and bowel control. It plays a key role in preventing incontinence, which can be a significant issue for many women, especially after childbirth or during menopause.

Second, the pelvic floor is integral to sexual health and satisfaction. It's involved in sexual function and can impact sensations during intercourse. A weakened or overly tight pelvic floor can lead to discomfort, pain, or reduced sensation.

Furthermore, during pregnancy and childbirth, the pelvic floor muscles stretch and can become weakened. This can lead to issues like prolapse, where the organs the pelvic floor supports can descend and cause discomfort or other health problems.

In my experience, pelvic floor health is not just a medical concern; it's deeply connected to a woman's quality of life. It affects physical activity, confidence, sexual well-being, and overall health, both physical and mental. Yet, it's often a neglected area in women's healthcare.

### What is Hyivy?

It's a unique, intelligent, and integrated pelvic rehabilitation system that addresses various pelvic health issues. Hyivy is an IoT (Internet of

Things) device at its core. It utilizes smart technology to gather data and provide feedback for better treatment and understanding pelvic health.

Hyivy consists of a therapeutic vaginal wand, which is modular and customizable to fit the specific needs of different users. This modularity allows various therapeutic modules to be attached, such as those for heat and cold therapy or automatic dilation. These modules address a range of pelvic floor dysfunctions by providing targeted treatments. For example, the heat and cold therapy module can help alleviate symptoms like pain or discomfort by providing soothing temperature treatments directly to the pelvic area.

One of Hyivy's most innovative aspects is its data collection and feedback mechanism. The device is equipped with sensors that can measure vital signs of the pelvic floor, like temperature, pressure, and moisture levels. This data is then processed to give users and their healthcare providers valuable insights into their pelvic health, allowing for more personalized and effective treatment plans.

It's particularly beneficial for women who are experiencing pelvic health issues due to various conditions such as menopause, childbirth, cancer treatments, surgeries, or pelvic floor disorders. It's also a valuable tool for women who have undergone gender reassignment surgery, as it addresses the specific needs and challenges they face in maintaining pelvic health.

In essence, Hyivy is a comprehensive platform that combines therapy, data collection, and personalized healthcare to improve the quality of life for women dealing with pelvic health issues. We are also excited to see other FemTech companies creating solutions to help prevent pelvic floor injury.

## Tracy MacNeal, CEO at Materna Medical

*Materna Medical specializes in addressing pelvic conditions in women; specifically, their products assist women with intimate health challenges and prevent pelvic injuries in childbirth. Episode 17 aired June 8, 2020.*

### What is pelvic organ prolapse?

Pelvic organ prolapse is a condition that occurs when the muscles and tissues supporting the pelvic organs (like the bladder, uterus, and rectum) become weak or loose. This weakening can cause one or more of these organs to drop or press into or out of the vagina. It's a condition that's more common than many realize, and it can significantly impact a woman's quality of life.

Depending on the organ involved, there are different types of pelvic organ prolapse. For example, if the bladder drops, it's known as a cystocele, and if the rectum bulges into the back wall of the vagina, it's called a rectocele. Prolapse often occurs because of childbirth, but it can also develop due to aging, menopause, or other factors that strain or weaken the pelvic floor muscles.

Symptoms can vary, but they often include discomfort or pressure in the pelvic area, difficulties with urination and bowel movements, and issues during sexual intercourse. It's essential to understand that prolapse is a common issue and that there are various treatment options available ranging from physical therapy to strengthen the pelvic floor muscles to surgical interventions in more severe cases.

Women experiencing any symptoms of prolapse should seek medical advice. Early intervention can significantly improve the management of the condition and the quality of life.

### Tell us about injuries during childbirth.

Childbirth-related injuries are more common than many people realize. The rates of injury can vary depending on several factors, including the type of delivery, the size of the baby, and the mother's health. However, it's important to note that a significant proportion of women experience some form of injury during childbirth. For instance, perineal tears, which are tears in the tissue between the vagina and anus, occur in about 90 percent of first-time vaginal births where the woman has not had a surgical cut (episiotomy).

There are different degrees of perineal tears, ranging from minor, which involves only the skin, to more severe tears that extend to the muscles and, in the most severe cases, to the anal sphincter and rectum. The treatment of these tears depends on their severity. Minor tears may heal on their own or with minimal stitching, while more severe ones require surgical repair and require a more extended recovery period.

The long-term consequences of childbirth-related injuries can vary. While many women recover with no lasting effects, some may experience ongoing symptoms such as incontinence, pelvic pain, or painful intercourse. Severe perineal tears can lead to complications like fecal incontinence or chronic pain if not properly managed. Women must receive appropriate care and follow-up after childbirth to address these injuries effectively.

Our flagship product in development is Materna Prep, a preventive device aimed at reducing the incidence of pelvic floor injuries during childbirth. The concept behind Prep is based on gently and safely preparing the birth canal for delivery. It's a mechanical device that provides a controlled stretch to the birth canal muscles, reducing the risk of tearing and other injuries that can occur during childbirth.

The development of Prep is grounded in extensive clinical research. Our goal is to provide a safe, effective, and noninvasive method for women to significantly reduce their risk of sustaining childbirth injuries. By addressing these injuries proactively, we can improve mothers' outcomes and reduce the long-term health complications associated with childbirth. It's exciting to see all the new innovations in pelvic floor health; even ancient devices like pessaries are being revamped.

## Derek Sham, MBA, Founder and CEO at Cosm Medical

*Cosm Medical's mission is to advance the field of female public health by modernizing outdated technology. They are innovating the pessary using ultrasound, AI, and 3D-printing technologies to create patient-specific solutions. Episode 182 aired September 26, 2022.*

### What is a pessary?

A pessary is one of the oldest medical devices, dating back around 4,000 years. It is a device placed inside the vagina to provide support for pelvic organs. It is commonly used in the treatment of pelvic floor disorders such as pelvic organ prolapse and urinary incontinence. Pessaries are quite common, with over ten million women globally using them.

They work by acting as a support structure within the vagina, like how a sports bra supports breasts. Different pessaries serve different purposes; some are used for organ prolapse, while others are designed for urinary incontinence. The effectiveness of a pessary depends on its type, fit, and the specific pelvic floor disorder it's addressing.

Pessaries are given to women primarily to provide nonsurgical treatment options for pelvic floor disorders. They offer an alternative to surgery, which can be invasive and has its own risks. Pessaries can be particularly beneficial for women who are not candidates for surgery, such as elderly women or those with certain medical conditions.

However, there are challenges in using pessaries. Traditional pessaries come in various shapes and sizes and are often fitted by trial and error, which can be uncomfortable and time-consuming for the patient. Long-term use of pessaries can lead to complications like tissue abrasion, infections, and vaginal discharge. Additionally, some types are not conducive to sexual activity or menstruation, requiring removal and reinsertion, which can be cumbersome for the user.

## What is Cosm Medical?

Cosm Medical is a pioneering company in digital gynecology focused on personalized care for women suffering from pelvic floor disorders. We are revolutionizing the pessary industry by leveraging cutting-edge technologies like ultrasound, artificial intelligence (AI), and 3D printing. Our goal is to bring pelvic floor health into the twenty-first century and improve the quality of life for women worldwide.

Our technology works by creating a more personalized and effective solution for pelvic floor disorders, such as pelvic organ prolapse and urinary incontinence. We developed a unique measurement technology to accurately scan and mold the female pelvic floor. Combined with AI-driven software, this data enables us to predict and create custom designs for each patient. These designs are then brought to life through 3D printing, resulting in patient-specific devices tailored to each woman's unique anatomy and needs.

What sets Cosm Medical apart is our unique business model. We are not just creating a medical device but developing a comprehensive digital gynecology platform. This approach allows us to continuously gather data, learn from each patient's experience, and refine our products. It's a model that benefits the individual patient and contributes to the broader understanding of pelvic floor health.

Additionally, we are adopting a revenue-sharing model similar to what's seen in other medical fields (like dentistry with Invisalign). This model is designed to be mutually beneficial for both healthcare providers and patients. It incentivizes healthcare providers to adopt our technology by offering them a share of the revenue, while patients receive more personalized and effective treatment. We believe this approach will encourage wider adoption and ultimately lead to better outcomes for women suffering from pelvic floor disorders.

## Missy Lavender, MBA, Founder and CEO at Renalis

*Renalis is an FDA-cleared prescription drug from Digital Therapeutics for the treatment of pelvic health disorders, including overactive bladder. Episode 216 aired July 5, 2023.*

### What is overactive bladder?

Overactive bladder (OAB) is a common condition that affects millions of individuals, characterized by a sudden, frequent, and often uncontrollable urge to urinate. It differs from stress urinary incontinence, which involves urine leakage during physical activities like coughing or sneezing. OAB occurs when the bladder muscles involuntarily contract, creating an urgent need to urinate, even if the bladder isn't full. These bladder spasms can disrupt daily life, leading to frequent bathroom visits and potentially affecting sleep and overall quality of life.

OAB can manifest in various ways. Some individuals experience dry overactive bladder, where they feel the urge to urinate urgently but don't necessarily leak urine. Others may have wet overactive bladder, where the urge is accompanied by urine leakage, known as urge incontinence.

The underlying causes of OAB are not entirely understood, but it's thought to be related to the bladder's muscles and nerves functioning improperly. Factors like age, obesity, and certain neurological conditions can increase the risk of developing OAB. For many, the onset of symptoms intensifies around menopause, likely due to hormonal changes, particularly the reduction in estrogen.

Treatment for OAB often begins with behavioral and lifestyle changes, such as bladder training, pelvic floor exercises, and dietary modifications to avoid bladder irritants like caffeine and alcohol. In some cases, medications, Botox injections, or even nerve stimulation therapies may be recommended. It's essential to consult a healthcare provider for proper diagnosis and to discuss the best treatment options for individual cases.

### How does Renalis work?

Renalis is a groundbreaking digital health platform that focuses on addressing pelvic health disorders, starting with OAB. At Renalis, we understand that managing OAB goes beyond just medical treatments; it's about empowering individuals with the knowledge and tools to take control of their bladder health.

Our key product, CeCe, is a digital therapeutic designed to deliver behavioral therapy through a smartphone or smart device. CeCe is like having a personal bladder health coach in your pocket. It guides users through educational modules and interactive exercises tailored to their needs and symptoms. The app collects data on bladder habits, symptoms, and lifestyle factors, allowing for a personalized and data-driven approach to managing OAB.

One of the core components of CeCe is its focus on bladder training and pelvic floor exercises. These exercises are crucial in strengthening the pelvic floor muscles, which can help reduce the urgency and frequency of urination. Additionally, CeCe provides strategies for urge suppression and lifestyle modifications, such as dietary changes, which can play a significant role in managing OAB symptoms.

Another innovative feature of CeCe is its emphasis on cognitive behavioral techniques. We recognize that OAB is not just a physical condition but also has psychological aspects. CeCe helps users develop coping strategies to manage the anxiety and stress that often accompany OAB, improving their overall quality of life.

Furthermore, Renalis is committed to ensuring that CeCe is evidence-based and clinically validated. We're pursuing FDA clearance for CeCe as a prescribed digital therapeutic, which means it will undergo rigorous testing and research to ensure its effectiveness and safety.

In summary, Renalis, through CeCe, provides a comprehensive, accessible, and user-friendly solution for individuals managing overactive bladders. It offers a holistic approach that combines medical, behavioral, and lifestyle interventions to effectively manage and improve bladder health.

* * *

In this chapter on pelvic floor health, the profound impact of pelvic floor disorders on women's lives is brought to light through narratives like Margaret's, a retired kindergarten teacher whose life was disrupted by urinary incontinence. This common issue among women, often exacerbated by childbirth and aging, underscores the critical importance of proper pelvic health management and the broader implications for physical and emotional well-being. Despite long-standing challenges in addressing these issues, advancements in medical and technological fields are providing new avenues for treatment and support. Innovations such as pelvic floor therapy and personalized medical devices are not only enhancing the understanding and management of pelvic floor disorders, but they are also empowering women to take control of their health with dignity and confidence. The chapter emphasizes the necessity for continued advocacy for better healthcare practices and policies that support women's health needs comprehensively, ensuring that future generations have better access to information and care regarding pelvic floor health.

# Chapter 10
# Menopause

**AS JADA STOOD POISED IN THE COURTROOM,** ready to address the judge, a role she had earned after years of relentless dedication at her law firm, a sudden, unwelcome heat engulfed her. At that moment, with the eyes of the court on her, the reality of menopause hit with its most notorious symptom—a hot flash. Sweat beaded across her forehead, the intense warmth threatening to undermine her composed exterior. *Oh please, not now,* she silently pleaded, feeling the temperature in the room soar to unbearable degrees. The judge's voice, asking if she was ready, seemed distant as she struggled to maintain professionalism. Grasping for control, Jada requested a brief recess, her voice steady despite the chaos erupting within her.

Hurrying to the sanctuary of the restroom, Jada splashed cool water on her face, trying to quell the fire that raged under her skin. The night before had been another battle with sleeplessness, courtesy of relentless hot flashes, and now, nine months into these symptoms, exhaustion had become a constant companion. Standing there, looking at her reflection marked by the signs of her struggle, Jada was acutely aware of the challenge menopause posed not just physically, but also in her ability to perform at the peak of her legal career. The thought of enduring this indefinitely was daunting. As she braced herself to return to the courtroom, she realized the necessity of finding a way to manage her symptoms effectively, lest they derail the hard-earned achievements of her storied career.

Menopause, a natural biological process, marks the end of a woman's menstrual cycle and fertility. It is a universal phenomenon among women, typically occurring between ages forty-five and fifty-five (average age is fifty-one), but its implications extend far beyond mere biology, touching upon cultural, societal, and economic spheres.[93,94]

Menopause is characterized by the cessation of menstruation, occurring twelve months after a woman's final natural ovulation cycle. The menopausal transition, or perimenopause, usually lasts seven years but can endure as long as fourteen years, starting in the early forties, and is influenced by race and ethnicity alongside various lifestyle factors. During this time, women may experience symptoms like hot flashes, sleep disturbances, mood fluctuations, and changes in their periods—including bleeding more or less than usual and more intermittently. Hot flashes can last between thirty seconds and ten minutes and happen several times an hour or just a couple of times a week and can even be strong enough to cause heavy sweating and cold shivering, causing women to wake up (referred to as night sweats). All these symptoms result from fluctuating levels of estrogen and progesterone, hormones produced by the ovaries. Interestingly, menopause is rare in the animal kingdom, documented only in humans, orcas, and short-finned pilot whales, suggesting its unique evolutionary significance.

Historically, menopause has been viewed through various lenses, often reflecting prevailing societal attitudes toward aging and female fertility. In ancient Greece, menopause was recognized as a natural cessation of menstruation, and it progressed with limited medical intervention. However, by the eighteenth century, this perspective started to shift, and over the next 300 years, menopause began to be medicalized and regarded as a disease requiring treatment. This medicalization paved the way for the development and popularization of hormone replacement therapy in the mid-twentieth century, despite the lack of understanding of its long-term effects, which would only come to light decades later.

Despite the prevalence and impact of menopause on women's health, there is a surprising lack of comprehensive education on the topic within medical schools. This gap in medical education leaves many healthcare providers ill-equipped to support women through the menopausal transition, contributing to the underdiagnosis and undertreatment of menopausal symptoms. Medical school students and OB-GYN residents in the US are not required to take any courses in peri/menopause. A national survey of program directors found only 31.3% of OB-GYN residential programs included a curriculum on menopause, underscoring the need for improved training and awareness.[95]

Cultural attitudes toward menopause vary significantly around the globe. In many Indigenous and traditional societies, menopause is revered as transitioning to a respected status of elder wisdom and leadership. Contrastingly, in Western societies, menopause is often viewed negatively, associated with aging and loss of fertility. This cultural dichotomy influences how women experience and perceive menopause, affecting their mental and emotional well-being during this transitional phase.

As women constitute an increasing proportion of the workforce and account for 45 percent of the paid workforce over fifty years old, menopause has emerged as a significant workplace issue.[96] Symptoms of menopause can adversely affect work performance and productivity, with four out of every ten women confirming this in the Biote Women in the Workplace survey.[97]

Menopause costs American women $1.8 billion in lost working time per year, as reported by the Mayo Clinic in 2023.[98] Research by the Mayo Clinic in Minnesota, Arizona, Florida, and Wisconsin also reported a greater proportion of adverse work outcomes related to menopausal symptoms for Black and Hispanic working women compared to White women. The Biote Women in the Workplace survey demonstrates that 17 percent of women have either quit a job or considered quitting due to menopause symptoms. In fact, half a million women between ages 55 to 64 leave the workforce due to menopause symptoms.[99] Despite this, 87 percent of women do not feel comfortable discussing their symptoms with employers, fearing stigma and discrimination.[100] Only 34 percent of respondents felt that people experiencing workplace challenges would receive support. This highlights the need for workplace policies and support systems that acknowledge and accommodate the unique needs of menopausal women, ensuring they can continue to contribute effectively to the workforce.[101]

Menopause is a complex and deeply personal experience that intersects with biology, culture, history, and economics. As society progresses, there is a growing recognition of the need to demystify menopause, improve medical education, and foster supportive environments, both medically and in the workplace. By addressing the challenges associated with menopause openly and proactively, we can empower women to navigate this transition with confidence and dignity, celebrating it not as an end but as a new chapter of life rich with potential.

Menopause is one of the fastest-growing verticals in women's health innovation, with 7 percent of all FemTech startups focused on addressing its most common and disruptive symptoms. In fact, 73 percent of menopause startups were founded in the last five years, making this one of the most recent verticals for FemTech innovation.[102, 103]

## Ann Garnier, Founder and CEO at Midday

*Midday is an app that leverages AI, sensor technology, and digital therapeutics to support women on their menopause journey. It uses personalized insights to illuminate what is happening physically and emotionally during menopause, providing the right intervention at the right time to manage menopause symptoms and promote healthy aging.*
*Episode 21 aired June 22, 2020.*

### How are menopause symptoms treated?

Menopause is associated with thirty-four different symptoms, which significantly impact various aspects of a woman's life. The prevalence and duration of these symptoms vary widely among women, but they commonly include hot flashes, night sweats, mood changes, fatigue, and changes in libido. These symptoms can affect a woman's professional life, relationships, and well-being.

We categorize treatments into three main areas for effective management: hormonal solutions, nonhormonal prescription-based solutions, and nonprescription alternative and complementary medicine interventions. Given the lack of training among general practitioners in this area, it's crucial for women to consult with healthcare providers trained in menopausal care to explore hormone therapy options. Additionally, lifestyle interventions are a pivotal aspect of managing menopause symptoms. Research suggests that lifestyle changes can significantly impact symptomatology.

Moreover, embracing technology and data-driven solutions is paramount. We're utilizing predictive algorithms to offer personalized plans based on clinically validated tools. This approach enhances symptom management and tailors interventions to each woman's unique needs.

Finally, investment in menopause research and technology is essential. Despite the increasing visibility of FemTech, investment in early stage companies focusing on menopause remains limited. A concerted effort toward funding and research is crucial for advancing care in this field, benefiting millions of women undergoing the menopause transition.

### How does menopause affect women of various ethnicities differently?

Menopause symptoms indeed vary across different ethnicities, a phenomenon underscored by significant research, including findings from the Study of Women's Health Across the Nation (SWAN). For example, Black women tend to experience moderate to severe hot flashes more frequently and for a longer duration compared to their counterparts. On the other hand, Japanese women, possibly due to dietary factors like high soy intake, often report milder symptoms or even a complete absence of hot flashes.

These variations suggest that genetic, dietary, and lifestyle factors contribute to how menopause symptoms manifest across different ethnic groups. Healthcare providers must recognize and incorporate these differences when advising on menopause management strategies. Tailoring treatments and lifestyle recommendations to reflect these variances can significantly improve the quality of care and outcomes for menopausal women from diverse backgrounds. Our company and others are leading the forefront of providing adequate care for menopausal women.

## Jannine Versi, Cofounder and CEO at Elektra Health

*Elektra Health is a next-generation healthcare platform for the tens of millions of women currently and soon to be navigating perimenopause and menopause. It provides access to one-on-one guidance to build a personalized plan that prioritizes evidence-based care.*
*Episode 63 aired November 16, 2020.*

### How are integrative and lifestyle-based approaches effective treatments for menopause?

Integrative and lifestyle-based approaches consider not just the physical symptoms but also the emotional, mental, and lifestyle aspects of a woman's life during menopause. Lifestyle modifications, including diet changes, regular physical activity, and stress management techniques such as mindfulness and yoga, can significantly impact the severity and frequency of menopausal symptoms.

For instance, dietary adjustments to include more phytoestrogens in foods like soy can help balance hormone levels naturally. Regular exercise improves cardiovascular health, bone density, mood, and weight management, which can be particularly beneficial as women navigate menopause. Additionally, stress-reducing practices such as meditation or deep-breathing exercises can alleviate symptoms like hot flashes and improve sleep quality.

The North American Menopause Society highlights that approximately forty million women are currently navigating through menopause in the United States alone. Yet, a significant gap exists in the training of healthcare providers, with only about 20 percent of OB-GYN residency programs covering menopause comprehensively. This lack of education leads to many women not receiving the care and support they need during this transition. Integrative and lifestyle-based approaches, therefore, offer a valuable and often underutilized avenue for treatment, emphasizing personalized care that addresses the whole person rather than a one-size-fits-all solution.

**Tell us about the history of hormone replacement therapy (HRT).**

The controversy around hormone replacement therapy (HRT) for menopause symptoms largely stems from the Women's Health Initiative (WHI) study published in 2002. This landmark study initially reported that HRT could lead to an increased risk of breast cancer, heart disease, strokes, and blood clots. The publication of these results caused widespread panic. It led to a significant decline in HRT prescriptions, with many women stopping their therapy abruptly and doctors becoming hesitant to prescribe it.

However, subsequent analyses and follow-up studies have nuanced these findings. It's been recognized that the WHI study's initial results were somewhat oversimplified. For instance, the study included women who were, on average, ten years past menopause, which is not the typical demographic for initiating HRT. The risks identified were primarily associated with older women and those using a specific combination of estrogen and progestin.

Further research indicated that HRT could be safe and beneficial for symptom relief in women who start treatment closer to the onset of menopause, typically within ten years. The benefits of HRT, such as relief from hot flashes, night sweats, and vaginal dryness, and potential protection against osteoporosis, were reiterated, especially when personalized to the individual's health profile and needs.

Despite the clarification and nuanced understanding of HRT's risks and benefits, skepticism and hesitancy persist. This attitude can be attributed to the initial scare and the ongoing debate in the public and among healthcare providers about the interpretation of the WHI study results. Luckily women who are still nervous to take HRT can hopefully still feel relief from their symptoms with new, natural products coming from the FemTech industry.

## Gwendolyn Floyd, Cofounder and CEO at Wile

*Wile manufactures plant-based supplements to support the hormonal and mental well-being of women aged forty and up. Wile combines clinical research with plant medicine to debunk and embrace adult women's hormonal influences and internal complexity.*
*Episode 139 aired November 1, 2021.*

**Is there a stigma around menopause? What can we do about it?**

There's a deep stigma around menopause, and it's rooted in societal perceptions of aging. This stigma is not only unwarranted but harmful, perpetuating silence and misunderstanding about a natural phase in a woman's life. The root of this issue lies in the lack of education and open dialogue. Many women enter perimenopause and menopause without understanding what's happening to their bodies, leading to confusion and sometimes fear.

Education and storytelling play pivotal roles in dismantling these stigmas. By openly discussing menopause and perimenopause, sharing experiences, and providing accurate information, we can normalize this stage of life, reducing fear and misinformation. Educational initiatives should start early, ensuring that both women and men understand women's health across all life stages.

Statistically, it's reported that nearly one in three women are either in perimenopause or postmenopause, yet the dialogue around this significant part of a woman's life remains hushed. Integrating menopause education into general health education can change narratives, empowering women to approach menopause with confidence rather than apprehension.

Moreover, storytelling, particularly from diverse voices, can illuminate how menopause affects women, highlighting that while some struggle, others may have newfound vitality. Stories can provide comfort, shared experiences, and even solutions that medical discussions sometimes overlook.

**What is Wile? Why did you start it?**

I started Wile because of my own challenging journey through early onset perimenopause. The realization of a profound lack of education, understanding, and support for women during this significant life phase propelled me. It's not just a company; it's a mission to shift the narrative around women's health, specifically around the transformative stages of perimenopause and menopause, from one of stigma and silence to one of empowerment and open dialogue.

At Wile, we recognize that nearly half of the population will experience menopause, yet the conversation and support surrounding it are woefully inadequate. Our products are designed to address this gap, offering plant-based, scientifically backed solutions that support women's bodies naturally. We've developed a range of supplements and tinctures tailored to women's specific needs and symptoms during perimenopause and beyond.

Our product lineup includes supplements aimed at hormonal balance, supporting menstrual regularity, managing symptoms associated with hot flashes and night sweats, and addressing stress, anxiety, and the unique metabolic changes during this phase of life. Each product is crafted with a blend of herbs and natural ingredients, chosen for their efficacy and historical use in supporting women's health.

We also offer a range of tinctures designed for real-time symptom relief, recognizing that perimenopause can present a roller coaster of symptoms that vary from day to day. These include formulations to help manage moments of intense stress or irritability, support mood and energy levels, and promote better sleep—all without relying on synthetic hormones or pharmaceuticals. These solutions are critical since menopause affects every aspect of a woman's life, from sleep to sex.

## Barb DePree, MD, Founder at MiddlesexMD

*Dr. Barb DePree, a practicing gynecologist for over thirty years, founded MiddlesexMD after witnessing the challenges women in perimenopause and beyond face regarding sexual pleasure. MiddlesexMD serves as a health resource, offering reliable information to narrow the pleasure gap within this age group. Episode 25 aired July 6, 2020.*

### How does menopause affect sexual wellness?

Menopause significantly impacts sexual wellness, affecting nearly 50 percent of women within five years of postmenopause with symptoms that are not resolved with over-the-counter products. This percentage escalates as time progresses. The importance of sexual satisfaction is underscored by research, indicating that it contributes an additional 15 to 20 percent to the value of relationships when it's positive. In contrast, dissatisfaction or the absence of sexual activity can adversely affect relationships by 50 to 70 percent.

It's noteworthy that 94 percent of American adults, encompassing both genders, believe that sexual satisfaction is crucial for a good quality of life. However, it's surprising that only 10 to 20 percent have ever broached this topic with a healthcare professional. This discrepancy highlights a significant unmet need, as discussions on sexual wellness are not commonly prioritized by healthcare providers, possibly due to time limitations or discomfort with the subject matter. This gap in communication and support spans across various life stages, emphasizing the necessity for more inclusive and open conversations on sexual health and satisfaction.

The primary and most consistent change associated with menopause is the consequence of the loss of estrogen. This hormonal shift has a direct impact on the vulva, vagina, and lower urinary tract, all areas with abundant estrogen receptors. Without estrogen, these tissues experience reduced blood supply, sensitivity, and elasticity, leading to narrower vaginal walls and increased dryness, fragility, and pain during sexual intercourse. Consequently, sex becomes less comfortable or even painful, prompting women to avoid it, which only exacerbates the discomfort over time.

Many women are unaware that these changes are directly linked to menopause, often attributing them to aging or other factors. This lack of awareness contributes to a significant quality-of-life issue, as sexual satisfaction is deemed an important aspect of life by a vast majority of

American adults. Yet, discussions around this topic with healthcare providers are rare, with many women believing there are no treatments available or fearing their concerns will be dismissed.

My mission with MiddlesexMD is to offer a safe, comfortable space for women to learn about and address the changes in sexual health that come with aging, particularly those related to menopause. The website aims to provide knowledge, resources, and products that can help alleviate these symptoms. From selecting the right lubricants and moisturizers to understanding the benefits of vibrators for maintaining blood flow and tissue health, MiddlesexMD seeks to empower women with the tools they need to maintain or regain their sexual health.

It's crucial to recognize that the conversation around menopause and sexual wellness should also include partners, as their understanding and support can significantly influence treatment success and relationship satisfaction. Addressing sexual wellness in the context of menopause requires a holistic approach, considering physical, emotional, and relational factors. Through education and open dialogue, we can support women in navigating these changes, ensuring they continue to enjoy fulfilling sexual relationships and overall well-being during menopause and beyond.

* * *

In the chapter on menopause, we delve into the complexities of this inevitable phase in a woman's life, bringing to light its profound effects not just biologically, but across cultural, societal, and economic layers. This chapter reveals how menopause, often shrouded in silence and stigma, transcends mere biological change, affecting millions with its multifaceted impacts. It underscores the critical need for broader education, better healthcare responses, and workplace policies that acknowledge and support women through this transition. By reframing menopause as an important aspect of women's health and advocating for systemic change, we empower women to manage their symptoms effectively and embrace this phase of life not as an end, but as a new beginning full of potential. As the discourse around menopause continues to evolve, the chapter calls for a shift in perception—from a taboo subject to an embraced natural stage of life—ensuring women are supported holistically through their menopausal journey.

# Chapter 11
# Cancer

**IN THE REALM OF ONCOLOGY,** a stark disparity exists between genders, with men facing a higher propensity for cancer, evidenced by a one-in-two lifetime risk compared to one in three for women.[104] Despite this, certain cancers disproportionately affect women, both in prevalence and mortality rates, and the funding for research into these cancers often does not reflect the severity of the impact.

Breast cancer stands as the most common cancer among women in the United States, aside from skin cancer.[105] It's a sobering reality that approximately one in eight women in the United States will confront invasive breast cancer over their lifetime.[106] Despite significant advances in treatment and awareness, breast cancer remains the second leading cause of cancer death in women, trailing only lung cancer.[107] This highlights a critical need for continued research and improved therapeutic strategies.

Lung cancer, traditionally associated with smoking, has emerged as a leading cause of cancer death among women, surpassing breast cancer in some statistics.[108] Alarmingly, lung cancer diagnoses in women have surged by 84 percent over the past four decades, a stark contrast to the 36 percent decline observed among men.[109] This trend, coupled with the fact that nonsmoking women are more than twice as likely to develop lung cancer as their smoking male counterparts, points to a critical gap in understanding and addressing this disease in women.[110] Moreover, the disparity in funding, with only 15 percent of the National Institutes of Health's lung cancer budget allocated to women-focused research, further exacerbates the issue.[111]

Cervical, endometrial, and ovarian cancers constitute major health concerns for women, with the human papillomavirus (HPV) being a significant risk factor for cervical cancer. Despite the availability of preventive measures like the HPV vaccination, these cancers continue to affect thousands of women annually. Research funding for gynecologic cancers—when normalized to years of life lost—ranks disappointingly low compared to other cancers such as prostate cancer, highlighting a glaring disparity in the allocation of resources.[112]

Recent studies have shed light on the pronounced sex disparities in the side effects of cancer treatments. Women are 34 percent more likely to experience severe side effects from therapies, including chemotherapy, immunotherapy, and targeted therapy.[113] The sex disparity in severe side effects was the most pronounced among patients receiving immunotherapy, with women having a nearly 50 percent increased risk of serious side effects compared with men.[114] This discrepancy underscores the urgent need for sex-specific research and treatment approaches to mitigate these adverse impacts on women undergoing cancer treatment.

The funding landscape for women's health research reveals a stark imbalance. Pharmaceutical companies dedicate a mere 4 percent of approximately $200 billion to healthcare research and development focusing on women's health.[115] Of the $8 billion dedicated to women's health, 75 percent of it is allocated to female cancer specifically.[116] This leaves just $2 billion to the rest of women's health. This disparity reflects what issues in women's health pharma is willing to invest in and which areas they are most comfortable funding versus conditions like endometriosis or vulvodynia.

It's not just the private sector that underfunds women's health research. A recent study of the funding of eighteen types of cancers by the National Cancer Institute found that gynecologic cancers (ovarian, cervical, uterine) ranked tenth, twelfth, and fourteenth, respectively, in funding normalized to years of life lost, whereas prostate cancer ranked first.[117]

The intersection of artificial intelligence (AI) and cancer research represents a burgeoning frontier with the potential to revolutionize diagnosis, treatment, and prognostication. Limitations have historically hampered the battle against cancers prevalent among women in early detection and personalized treatment approaches. However, AI's advent is poised to usher in a new era of precision medicine, marked by enhanced detection accuracy and a more nuanced understanding of individual patient profiles.

Breast cancer has become a focal point for AI applications. While effective, traditional screening methods have limitations, including false positives and the potential for overdiagnosis, AI algorithms are showing promising results in identifying subtle signs of breast cancer in mammograms with a precision that rivals—and in some instances surpasses—human radiologists. A recent study published in *Radiology* shows that five AI-based algorithms can predict the five-year risk of breast cancer based on the mammogram and clinical factors of the patient.[118] This is the first time AI has predicted the long-term risk of cancer and could be a critical tool in reducing breast cancer deaths. The predictions were statistically significantly more accurate than the Breast Cancer Surveillance Consortium (BCSC) risk model, which is the tool relied on by healthcare professionals to calculate a female patient's risk of breast cancer within the next five years.

Researchers found that AI algorithms discriminate breast cancer risk significantly better and can predict the future risk of cancer for up to five years when no cancer is clinically detected in mammography. The results showed that AI predicted up to 28 percent of cancers versus 21 percent with BCSC.[119] These are substantial and clinically meaningful improvements in prediction. These AI-driven tools are not merely technological novelties but lifelines that could significantly lower mortality rates through early detection and intervention.

Unfortunately, the eradication of late-stage breast cancer depends on screening and access to healthcare. In 2019, only 67.5 percent of women over forty in the US had had a mammogram in the previous two years, with non-Hispanic Asian women the least likely of all groups to get a mammogram (64 percent).[120] One of the most significant barriers to screening is health insurance with only 42 percent of uninsured women having had a mammogram within the last two years.[121]

Predictive AI should also be used to locate and advocate for the women who miss mammograms. Can predictive AI identify who will most likely miss their mammogram and why? Can it tell us which programs would benefit specific communities most, such as providing free transportation versus free childcare at the clinic? A task force for these individuals could allow for more effective programs with consistently higher rates of screening and, thereby, significantly fewer cases of breast cancer in a community.

AI's role extends the entire cancer care continuum. In digital pathology, AI algorithms are being deployed to scrutinize tissue samples, enabling pathologists to detect abnormalities quickly and accurately. This capability is particularly crucial for cancers like ovarian and cervical, where early detection can dramatically affect outcomes. By parsing through vast datasets and identifying patterns imperceptible to the human eye, AI is enhancing our understanding of cancer's molecular underpinnings, paving the way for personalized treatment regimens tailored to an individual's genetic makeup. As we navigate this complex landscape, the goal remains clear: to improve outcomes and quality of life for women facing cancer, ensuring that they are not left behind in the global fight against this pervasive disease. Let's see how cancer organizations and FemTech are taking a stand on cancer for women.

## Suzanne Stone, CEO at LIVESTRONG

*LIVESTRONG is an organization that helps cancer survivors and their loved ones improve their quality of life. They believe in putting the survivor first and have created tools and resources to help ease the challenges of a cancer diagnosis. Episode 58 aired October 28, 2020.*

### Why do women need to consider their fertility before receiving treatment for cancer?

Treatments like chemotherapy and radiation can significantly impact their ability to conceive in the future. These treatments can damage eggs, affect the ovaries, and lead to conditions like premature ovarian failure, making it difficult or impossible to have biological children later on. Recognizing this, it's crucial for women of childbearing age who are diagnosed with cancer to explore fertility preservation options before starting their treatment.

Available options for fertility preservation include egg or embryo freezing, where eggs are harvested and either frozen unfertilized (egg freezing) or fertilized with a partner's or donor's sperm and then frozen (embryo freezing). This process must be done before beginning cancer treatment to ensure the eggs are not exposed to any damaging effects. Additionally, for some types of cancer, ovarian tissue freezing might be an option, where ovarian tissue is removed and reimplanted after treatment. However, this is less common and considered more experimental.

LIVESTRONG supports those facing these decisions by providing access to discounted fertility preservation services and medication through partnerships with over 730 clinics and pharmaceutical companies. This initiative reflects the importance of addressing the fertility impacts of cancer treatment, emphasizing the need for informed decision-making and access to preservation options for those wishing to have children in the future.

## What are the long-term consequences of receiving cancer treatment?

Cancer treatments, while lifesaving, can carry long-term consequences that profoundly impact survivors' quality of life. These effects vary widely among individuals but often include physical, emotional, and psychological challenges. For women, these consequences can be uniquely significant, touching on aspects of reproductive health, mental well-being, and the ability to perform daily activities.

One of the most critical, long-term effects for many women is on fertility, which we just discussed. Moreover, treatments can induce early menopause, bringing its suite of symptoms like hot flashes, mood swings, and increased risk of osteoporosis, further complicating a survivor's recovery journey. Physical changes, including weight gain, lymphedema, and changes in libido and sexual function, can also profoundly affect a woman's body image and self-esteem, potentially leading to long-term psychological effects, including anxiety, depression, and PTSD, particularly given the fear of recurrence that many survivors face.

Solutions have been developed to address these diverse and complex needs focusing on holistic recovery, encompassing physical and emotional rehabilitation. Programs like LIVESTRONG at the YMCA offer cancer survivors personalized exercise regimens to help rebuild strength and endurance. Additionally, LIVESTRONG's fertility preservation program provides discounted services and medication for those wishing to safeguard their ability to have children post-treatment.

Mental health support is equally crucial, with resources available through counseling and support groups tailored explicitly to cancer survivors, helping them navigate the emotional aftermath of their experience. Initiatives like the VitalHearts and Wonders & Worries programs focus on the secondary trauma experienced by healthcare providers and the children of those diagnosed with cancer, respectively, acknowledging the wide-reaching impact of the disease.

## Breast Cancer

### Fazila Seker, PhD, Cofounder and Former CEO at MOLLI Surgical

*MOLLI Surgical has developed a device that creates a better treatment journey for breast cancer patients. The device is a cutting-edge magnetic technology that shows surgeons where to remove tissue inside the breast, either a for lumpectomy to test for cancer or to remove a cancerous mass. Episode 128 aired August 9, 2021.*

#### What is a lumpectomy?

A lumpectomy, also known as breast-conserving surgery, is a procedure for removing cancer or other abnormal tissue from the breast. Women with early stage breast cancer often choose it because it allows them to keep most of their breast tissue. The surgery involves removing the tumor and a small margin of surrounding healthy tissue, offering an alternative to mastectomy, where the entire breast is removed.

This choice of surgery depends on various factors, including the size and location of the tumor, the breast's size, and the patient's personal preference. It's crucial for the decision to be made in consultation with a healthcare provider, considering all the potential risks and benefits. The primary goal of a lumpectomy is to remove cancer while conserving as much of the breast as possible, providing a balance between effective cancer treatment and quality of life post-surgery.

Following the surgery, patients usually undergo radiation therapy to eliminate any remaining cancer cells, reducing the risk of recurrence. The approach to lumpectomies continues to evolve, with ongoing research aimed at improving surgical techniques, minimizing side effects, and enhancing cosmetic outcomes, ensuring women have access to safe and effective breast-conserving options.

#### What is MOLLI Surgical?

Over 60 percent of breast tumors are so minuscule that they measure fewer than ten millimeters, making them virtually imperceptible by touch.

The conventional method for surgeons to locate and remove these small tumors involves a somewhat antiquated practice that MOLLI seeks to revolutionize.

MOLLI Surgical is replacing the outdated, uncomfortable wire localization method traditionally used during lumpectomies. Our technology centers around a tiny, magnetically detectable, marker, roughly the size of a grain of rice, precisely placed in or near the tumor before surgery. This marker, known as the MOLLI Marker, is detected during surgery with a handheld device, guiding surgeons directly to the tumor with remarkable accuracy.

The reason for developing MOLLI Surgical and moving away from the wire technique stems from the significant discomfort and logistic complications of wire localization. Traditionally, a wire is inserted into the breast on the day of surgery to mark the tumor's location, often causing discomfort for the patient and imposing strict logistic constraints on surgical scheduling. This method, while effective, is far from ideal in terms of patient experience and surgical efficiency.

MOLLI Surgical presents a vastly improved alternative, significantly enhancing the patient experience and the healthcare system's efficiency. From a patient's perspective, the MOLLI Marker is inserted in a minimally invasive procedure that can occur well before the surgery date, eliminating the discomfort and anxiety associated with wire localization. This flexibility also allows patients to better manage their schedules and reduces their time in the hospital, contributing to a more positive overall experience.

From a healthcare system standpoint, MOLLI Surgical offers several benefits. Allowing more flexible scheduling optimizes operating room utilization and reduces the bottleneck effect often seen with day-of-surgery wire placements. Furthermore, the precision of the MOLLI Marker can potentially lead to more effective tumor removal, possibly reducing the need for follow-up surgeries and, consequently, the overall cost of breast cancer treatment. MOLLI is dedicated to helping women receive the care they need when a small tumor is caught early because many complications can occur in women who have to undergo mastectomies and reconstructive surgeries.

## Kristen Carbone, Founder and CEO at Brilliantly

*Brilliantly is a company improving the lives of women who have been impacted by breast cancer. It has recently launched Brilliantly Warm, its first wearable designed for women who have had implant reconstruction after a mastectomy and feel constantly cold.*
*Episode 82 aired January 19, 2021.*

### Why did you start Brilliantly?

My journey was deeply personal and propelled by my own experiences and observations within the breast cancer community. My mother's battle with metastatic breast cancer and my subsequent preventive mastectomy, due to the high-risk factors identified in my own health, laid the foundation for my foray into women's health innovation. This decision, while lifesaving, introduced me to a myriad of post-surgical challenges that were largely unaddressed by the medical community, particularly the persistent and uncomfortable coldness experienced due to the implants.

This coldness, a seemingly minor yet pervasive issue, is emblematic of a larger problem faced by cancer survivors: the minimization of their post-treatment symptoms and quality-of-life concerns. The medical journey doesn't conclude with survival; for many, it's where the complexities of living with the aftermath begin. The silence around these issues, coupled with societal pressure to feel perpetually grateful for survival, often leaves women isolated in their struggles, hesitant to voice their discomfort or seek solutions.

Brilliantly was born out of a necessity to address not just the physical discomfort but to also challenge the narrative that surviving cancer is the end of the journey. The issue of feeling perpetually cold due to breast implants is more common than publicly acknowledged, affecting a significant portion of women who have undergone mastectomies and reconstruction. Through extensive conversations and research, it became evident that this was not a unique experience but a widespread concern that had been largely ignored.

The dismissal of cancer survivors' symptoms post-treatment is reflective of a broader societal and medical inclination to prioritize survival over the quality of post-survival life. This oversight not only diminishes the lived experiences of survivors but also impedes the development of holistic care approaches that address the entirety of a patient's health, including their physical comfort, mental well-being, and emotional resilience post-cancer.

The Brilliantly device operates on a simple yet effective principle. It's a noninvasive, wearable piece that fits snugly around the chest, much like a standard piece of clothing or accessory. Using safe, low-level heat generated by a battery-powered element, it delivers consistent, gentle warmth directly to the area of the breast implants. The heat is carefully regulated to ensure it provides comfort without risking overheating or discomfort.

This technology is particularly beneficial in cooler climates or environments where the discrepancy between the body's natural temperature and the saline implants becomes more pronounced. By maintaining a steadier, more body-similar temperature, the device helps women feel more comfortable and confident in their daily lives.

### Why are women with reconstructed breasts feeling cold?

Saline implants can conduct heat differently from the body's natural tissues. Unlike fat and glandular tissue that comprise a natural breast, saline does not generate heat. Because saline has a high thermal conductivity, it can cause the implants to feel cold, especially in cooler environments.

The body's natural tissues can regulate temperature through blood flow and metabolic activity, which implants lack. This difference in thermal properties between the saline solution inside the implants and the body's tissues can lead to a noticeable sensation of coldness. I discovered that approximately 75 percent of women postmastectomy are bothered by the cold, with varying levels of discomfort.

Although I am passionate about supporting cancer survivors, I applaud the innovators creating solutions to predict and prevent breast cancer from the start.

## Kaitlin Christine, Founder and CEO at Gabbi

*Gabbi has a revolutionary breast cancer risk assessment and early detection solution delivering immediate, accurate results for women of all ages and all ethnicities. Episode 114 aired May 11, 2021.*

### What is Gabbi? Why did you start it?

It all began in my senior year of college, amid my passion for theater and creative expression, when my mother's breast cancer diagnosis shook my world. The severity of her condition compelled me to leave college and become her full-time caregiver. Tragically, just eight months later, she passed away. This pivotal moment reshaped my entire outlook and career trajectory.

In the wake of my mother's death and facing my own breast health scare, I encountered significant challenges within the healthcare system. Despite having symptoms, I struggled to be taken seriously by healthcare professionals, an experience that highlighted systemic failings in women's healthcare. This battle wasn't just personal; it revealed a widespread issue affecting countless women who are often dismissed, underestimated, and inadequately informed about their health risks and options.

Gabbi emerged from a profound need to provide women with the knowledge, tools, and support necessary to navigate their health proactively. By leveraging technology, Gabbi aims to demystify healthcare, offering a trusted digital companion that guides women through their health concerns, educates them about their risks, and equips them with actionable insights tailored to their unique health profiles.

This risk assessment tool is grounded in healthcare models employed for women over twenty-five years. However, these models have primarily been confined to clinical settings within academia or health systems, rendering them inaccessible to the women they aim to benefit. Despite being recognized as standard care, only 1 percent of physicians incorporate these models into patient assessments. A significant drawback of these models is their limited applicability, primarily catering to White women aged thirty-five and above. To address this gap, we've developed a proprietary model capable of evaluating the lifetime risk for any woman, irrespective of age or ethnicity.

While the awareness of breast cancer affecting one in eight women is widespread, the association often ends with the color pink. Little action, tools, or advancements in early detection have been implemented. It seems as if mere awareness is considered sufficient, or perhaps the perception persists that breast cancer primarily impacts older women, specifically those aged fifty and above—a misconception we seek to dispel. Our ongoing pilot program with a health insurance company reaffirms our belief that breast cancer is prevalent in women under fifty, constituting 30 percent of diagnoses. For those not nearing fifty, mammograms may not be on their radar. The continued reliance on outdated screening mechanisms, especially in women's healthcare, where entry barriers are high, exacerbates the issue.

### What challenges do women face in getting a breast cancer diagnosis?

One of the critical barriers that women encounter is the challenge of being believed and taken seriously by healthcare professionals. There's a troubling trend of women's concerns being dismissed or minimized, especially when they report symptoms or express anxieties about their breast health. This skepticism from doctors can delay essential diagnostic tests like mammograms or biopsies, which are pivotal in detecting breast cancer at an early stage.

Our platform encourages women to document their symptoms meticulously, providing them with a concrete record of their health concerns to present to their doctors. This documentation can be instrumental in ensuring their concerns are taken seriously, facilitating a more productive dialogue with healthcare providers. By equipping women with accurate information and tools to articulate their experiences clearly, Gabbi aims to bridge the gap between patient concerns and professional medical advice, ensuring women receive the attention and care they deserve, right from the onset of symptoms.

## Cervical Cancer

### Molly Broache, MSN, WHNP, Associate Director at BD Integrated Diagnostic Solutions

*BD is one of the largest global medical technology companies in the world and is advancing the world of health by improving medical discovery, diagnostics, and the delivery of care. The company supports the heroes on the front lines of healthcare by developing innovative technology, services, and solutions that help advance both clinical therapy for patients and clinical processes for healthcare providers.*
*Episode 173 aired July 25, 2022.*

## What is HPV? How does it cause cervical cancer?

HPV, or human papillomavirus, is a group of viruses that includes more than one-hundred different strains or types. Over forty of these viruses are sexually transmitted and can infect the genital area of men and women. These include the skin of the penis, vulva, or anus, and the linings of the vagina, cervix, or rectum. Most people who become infected with HPV do not even know they have it.

Certain types of HPV are referred to as "high-risk" types because they are strongly associated with cancers, including types 16 and 18, which together account for approximately 70 percent of cervical cancer cases. An infection with high-risk HPV types can lead to the growth of abnormal cells on the cervix, known as dysplasia. Over time, these abnormal cells can develop into cancer if they are not detected and treated early. The transformation from a normal cervical cell into a cancerous cell is usually a slow process that can take several years, but it can sometimes happen more quickly. Low-risk types of HPV can also cause genital warts and respiratory papillomatosis, a rare condition where warts grow in the throat.

The prevalence of HPV poses a significant challenge, often referred to by my colleague as the common cold of STIs. Practically everyone who has been sexually active may have had some form of HPV infection. While screening very young women for cervical cancer with an HPV test is not recommended due to the body's typical clearance of the virus in one to two years, screenings should be considered if there are persistent infections. Notably, there are clear guidelines for females in cases of abnormal cells or a positive HPV test, but the absence of similar guidelines for males limits clinical utility. Establishing comprehensive guidelines for interpreting and acting on positive results in males could enhance the commercialization and wider approval of HPV tests.

To prevent HPV-related cancers, vaccines are available that protect against the most common high-risk types of HPV. These vaccines are most effective when given before an individual becomes sexually active. Screening for cervical cancer through Pap tests and HPV tests can also help detect changes in the cervix early before cancer develops. HPV tests are particularly important because they can identify the presence of high-risk HPV types that are most likely to cause cervical cancer.

### What test has BD developed?

BD has developed BD Onclarity™, the first FDA-approved HPV assay that reports six HPV strains individually, providing a more precise, accurate way to measure a woman's risk for developing cervical pre-cancer by showing results for an extended set of individual HPV strains and enabling those strains to be tracked over time. The most important determinant of cervical cancer risk in women who test positive for HPV is type-specific HPV persistence.

In essence, BD's cervical cancer screening test supports the shift toward more personalized and proactive healthcare. Through this test, BD aims to empower healthcare providers, improve patient outcomes, and ultimately, reduce the global burden of cervical cancer.

## Teo Tijerina, Founder and CEO at Hera Diagnostics

*Hera Diagnostics is a cancer diagnostics startup focusing on marketing a cervical cancer screening tool. The product is Herafem, a device used at the point of care that provides immediate results and a much more comfortable patient experience. Episode 73 aired December 21, 2020.*

### What is a Pap smear?

A Pap smear is a medical test that collects cells from the cervix to detect cervical cancer and precancerous conditions. Traditional Pap smears are less useful for women in rural areas for several reasons. First, traditional Pap smears have a lower sensitivity and can miss many cases of cervical cancer. In Mexico, sensitivities as low as 35 percent have been observed, making the test unreliable. Additionally, conducting and analyzing traditional Pap smears is complex, involving collecting cells, sending them to a laboratory, and waiting for results, which can take weeks or even months. This delay is problematic, especially in rural areas with limited access to healthcare facilities and specialists. Furthermore, when attempting to communicate results, it was found that about half of the women did not show up to receive their test results, highlighting a significant gap in the follow-up and treatment process. The lack of immediate, accurate testing, and the logistic challenges in reaching and following up with patients in remote areas, underscore the need for a more efficient, reliable, and accessible method for cervical cancer screening.

**What is Hera Diagnostics creating? Why is it uniquely useful for women in rural areas?**

The Hera Diagnostics tool is a transformative approach to cervical cancer detection, particularly vital in rural settings where traditional healthcare services may be scarce. Unlike the conventional Pap smear that requires laboratory analysis and faces challenges in accuracy and infrastructure, Hera Diagnostics operates through a technologically advanced method. It uses optical spectroscopy and electrical impedance to analyze cellular changes directly at the point of care. Herafem leverages a critical insight into the nature of cancerous versus noncancerous cells—specifically, their distinct electrical conductivity properties. By applying a minor electrical current to cervical cells via a specialized wand, Hera can monitor how these cells respond differently to the current.

Additionally, in regions like Latin America, HPV infection poses unique challenges due to the prevalence of HPV strains not covered by the most common vaccines. Our diagnostic device plays a crucial role in these scenarios by identifying cervical precancerous lesions early, irrespective of the HPV strain. This is particularly important because the HPV vaccine's effectiveness can vary based on the geographic and strain-specific prevalence of the virus. By providing a reliable screening method, Hera Diagnostics supports the early detection and prevention strategy for cervical cancer, complementing HPV vaccination programs and addressing the gaps where vaccines may not offer complete protection against locally prevalent strains.

The prevention of cervical cancer is critical when you realize the potential negative consequences of needing radiation.

## Julie Hakim, MD, Pediatric and Adolescent Gynecology Physician and Researcher at Baylor College of Medicine

*Dr. Julie Hakim is developing the first vaginal medical device explicitly designed to help vaginas heal following surgery and radiation treatments. The stent prevents complications from vaginal fibrosis after surgeries addressing reproductive anomalies and radiation treatment for gynecological cancers. Episode 2 aired April 6, 2020.*

## How does radiation therapy affect the vagina?

Radiation therapy, a standard treatment for various cancers, including those in the pelvic region, can lead to significant scarring in the vagina. This scarring, or vaginal stenosis, occurs because radiation damages not only the cancer cells but also the healthy tissue, leading to inflammation, reduced elasticity, and ultimately, fibrosis or scarring of the vaginal walls.

The consequences of this scarring are profound and multifaceted. First, it can lead to a significant decrease in quality of life due to pain, discomfort, and the loss of vaginal function, which includes painful intercourse, a condition known as dyspareunia. This not only affects physical health but also emotional well-being and intimate relationships. Moreover, vaginal stenosis can complicate or entirely prevent necessary medical examinations, like Pap smears, thereby impacting ongoing health surveillance and the ability to detect other conditions.

In terms of prevalence, while exact statistics can vary, the incidence of vaginal stenosis post-radiation therapy is reported to be high, with estimates suggesting that a significant portion of women receiving pelvic radiation will experience some degree of vaginal scarring. This underscores the importance of proactive measures, both for prevention and management, including the use of vaginal dilators as part of a post-treatment care regimen to maintain vaginal elasticity and function.

The broader implications of these statistics highlight a critical gap in patient care and education. There's a need for healthcare providers to not only inform patients about the potential side effects of radiation therapy including the risk of vaginal scarring but also to provide comprehensive support for managing these side effects. This includes offering resources, guidance on the use of vaginal dilators, and access to sexual health and pelvic floor specialists who can assist in managing and mitigating the impact of vaginal stenosis.

## What is a vaginal stent?

A vaginal stent is essentially a medical device designed to keep the vaginal canal open and support its healing process after surgery or radiation therapy. A well-designed vaginal stent could help prevent these issues by maintaining the structural integrity of the vagina during the healing process, reducing the risk of scarring and stenosis.

As of now, there's a significant gap in the market for an effective and specifically designed vaginal stent. The existing solutions are often make-shift, using materials not initially intended for this purpose, such as modified surgical gloves or other rudimentary devices. This gap exists partly due to historical oversight, under-prioritization of women's health issues in medical device development, and a need for more focused research and investment in this area.

By keeping the vaginal tissue supported and the canal at an appropriate width, a vaginal stent would not only aid in the physical recovery process but also have a profound impact on the patient's quality of life post-treatment. It addresses a critical but often overlooked aspect of recovery and represents a much-needed innovation in post-surgical and post-radiation therapy care for women.

The development of such a device would require a concerted effort from the medical community, including researchers, device manufacturers, and healthcare providers, to recognize the importance of this issue and allocate the necessary resources toward creating a solution. It's about time that the healthcare industry prioritizes and addresses the unique needs of women's health with the seriousness and dedication women deserve.

## Ovarian Cancer

### Oriana Papin-Zoghbi, Cofounder and CEO at AOA

*AOA's mission is to bring to market an accurate, early stage ovarian cancer diagnostic test that will improve clinical practice, help reduce patient mortality, and deliver cost savings to payers. Episode 120 aired June 14, 2021.*

#### What are the symptoms of ovarian cancer?

Ovarian cancer, often termed *the silent killer*, presents with symptoms that are easily mistaken for more benign conditions. Symptoms include bloating, pelvic or abdominal pain, feeling full quickly or having trouble eating, and urinary symptoms like urgency or frequency. Because these symptoms overlap with common gastrointestinal and urinary tract issues, they don't immediately raise alarms for ovarian cancer. This ambiguity, combined with the absence of effective early detection tests, like mammograms for breast cancer, results in most women being diagnosed at advanced stages when the disease has spread beyond the ovaries. Late-stage diagnosis significantly complicates treatment and reduces survival rates. Both healthcare professionals and women must recognize these symptoms early and consider ovarian cancer as a potential cause, especially if symptoms persist or worsen. Our goal is to enhance awareness and develop better screening methods to catch ovarian cancer earlier, ultimately improving outcomes for women worldwide.

Ovarian cancer risk is one in seven or eight women, and the primary challenges lie in the nonspecific symptoms and the absence of a diagnostic test. Ovarian cancer symptoms such as excessive bloating, changes in bowel movements, bleeding, and abdominal pain are often dismissed due to their commonality. The lack of belief in symptoms and the absence of a diagnostic test pose a significant hurdle.

Presently, there is no mammogram or PET scan for detection, and if a mass is under 1.5 centimeters (about 0.59 in), it won't appear on ultrasound. The only test used is the CA-125 test, approved for monitoring but not diagnosing ovarian cancer. Unfortunately, the diagnostic process involves exploratory biopsy surgery, which carries a high risk of ovarian loss, even if the cancer is not present.

With 80 percent of women diagnosed at stages 3 and 4, the survival rate is a mere 28 percent, highlighting the urgency for early detection. Black populations in the United States face higher incidence rates of ovarian cancer, making it a prevalent concern. The current state of ovarian cancer diagnosis is critical, with many women diagnosed at advanced stages and with limited access to specialized care, emphasizing the need for comprehensive and accessible diagnostic solutions.

### What test are you developing? What are the challenges of making a novel women's health diagnostic test?

We're developing a groundbreaking diagnostic test aimed at the early detection of ovarian cancer. The challenge with ovarian cancer is its nonspecific symptoms and the current lack of a reliable diagnostic tool. This ambiguity in symptoms often leads to late diagnosis, significantly reducing survival rates. Our test is designed to overcome these challenges by identifying specific biomarkers associated with ovarian cancer through a simple blood test. This not only aids in early detection but also eliminates the need for invasive procedures commonly used for diagnosis.

Developing a new diagnostic test involves navigating a complex landscape of regulatory, clinical, and market challenges. One of the primary hurdles is establishing a billing code, which is crucial for ensuring that insurance providers can reimburse for the test. Without this, achieving widespread adoption is challenging, regardless of the test's clinical value.

Conducting clinical studies is another significant barrier. These studies require substantial financial resources, time, and the ability to enroll sufficient participants to validate the test's efficacy and safety comprehensively. This process is critical for gaining regulatory approval and convincing the medical community of the test's utility.

Finally, updating medical guidelines to include a new test is a lengthy process that involves demonstrating the test's superiority or complementary value to existing standards of care. It requires engaging with and convincing numerous stakeholders, including medical professional societies, about the test's benefits. These challenges underscore the importance of not just innovation in the medical field, but also persistence and strategic navigation of the healthcare ecosystem to effectively bring new solutions to patients. There are only a few companies out there creating tests to help navigate ovarian masses and cancer.

## Nicole Sandford, Aspira Women's Health

*Aspira Women's Health aims to improve outcomes for those diagnosed with ovarian cancer with better detection and risk assessment. Their mission is to develop AI-powered diagnostic tools that improve gynecological health outcomes. Episode 229 aired February 28, 2024.*

### Tell us about ovarian masses.

Ovarian masses are a significant concern in women's health due to their potential to be benign or malignant. These masses can form for various reasons, including because of conditions like endometriosis or ovarian cysts. They are surprisingly common, affecting a considerable number of women at some point in their lives. In the United States, over 200,000 women undergo surgery for adnexal masses annually, though only about 10 percent of these cases are found to be ovarian cancer.[122] The critical challenge with ovarian masses lies in accurately diagnosing their nature, as the implications for treatment and prognosis differ vastly between benign and malignant cases.

Statistics indicate that while most ovarian masses are benign, the presence of a mass can significantly increase the anxiety and uncertainty for the patient. Early detection and accurate risk assessment are crucial for effective management. Advances in diagnostic technologies, such as the development of blood tests for ovarian cancer risk assessment, have been game-changer in this field. These tests provide a noninvasive method to help physicians make informed decisions regarding the need for surgery and the type of surgical intervention required, based on the likelihood of malignancy.

The goal is to improve outcomes by ensuring that women with high-risk masses receive prompt and appropriate treatment, while those with low-risk masses avoid unnecessary surgery. This approach not only has the potential to save lives by catching malignant cases early but also reduces the physical and emotional burden on women who would otherwise undergo unnecessary surgical procedures.

## What blood test has Aspira developed?

Aspira Women's Health has developed groundbreaking blood tests specifically designed to help in the early detection risk assessment of ovarian cancer for women with adnexal masses. This test works by analyzing specific biomarkers in the blood that are associated with ovarian cancer. By evaluating these biomarkers, the test can help assess the risk of ovarian cancer even in its early stages, when treatment is most effective. Doctors might use this test, along with other clinical assessments, for patients with adnexal masses planned for surgical intervention. It's particularly useful because it offers a noninvasive, accessible option for precise ovarian cancer risk assessment, which is crucial in improving outcomes for ovarian cancer patients. Aspira WH aims to provide women, especially those who may not have easy access to specialized healthcare services, with a reliable risk assessment tool, thereby significantly impacting their health and well-being.

* * *

In the chapter on cancer in women, we uncover the stark realities and unique challenges faced by women across the spectrum of cancer types, particularly those that affect them disproportionately. It also addresses the failure to meet the needs of women less advantaged. Despite advances in healthcare, there remains a persistent gap in research funding and understanding of cancers that primarily affect women, such as breast, lung, and gynecological cancers. This disparity not only hampers the development of targeted treatments but also deepens the impact on women's lives, emphasizing the urgent need for a more equitable approach in medical research and healthcare delivery. As we navigate the complexities of cancer in women, the chapter calls for enhanced awareness, improved funding for research, and better access to personalized treatments that consider the unique biological differences of women. By addressing these needs, we can ensure that women facing cancer receive the best possible care and support, ultimately improving outcomes and quality of life. This chapter sheds light on the hardships and celebrates the strides in technology and medicine that promise a more hopeful future for women battling cancer.

# Chapter 12
# Mental Health

**SOPHIE, A VIBRANT WOMAN IN HER MID-TWENTIES,** had always accepted the severe emotional turbulence she experienced just before her period as a normal facet of being a woman. Every month, like clockwork, three days before her menstruation, she would plunge into a deep depression. Her emotions weren't just typical premenstrual symptoms; they were overwhelming and crippling, leaving her sobbing uncontrollably and unable to get out of bed, sometimes even grappling with suicidal thoughts. Despite her struggle, whenever she reached out to friends or family, their responses were dismissive, equating her intense feelings with the common mood swings associated with menstrual cycles. This only reinforced her belief that her experience was just an extreme version of what everyone else went through, so she continued to suffer in silence, assuming she just needed to manage better.

It wasn't until Sophie's new roommate, Jenna, witnessed one of her episodes that the severity of the situation was truly acknowledged. Jenna, having never seen such profound despair tied to premenstrual symptoms, expressed concern and suggested that what Sophie was experiencing might be beyond typical premenstrual syndrome. This external validation was a revelation for Sophie; it was the first time someone recognized the gravity of her distress and did not normalize it as just part of the menstrual cycle. Encouraged by Jenna's concern and support, Sophie felt empowered to seek professional help. This decision led her to a diagnosis of premenstrual dysphoric disorder (PMDD), a severe form of premenstrual syndrome that was the root of her monthly emotional upheavals. Finally understanding the nature of her symptoms, Sophie began appropriate treatment, hopeful for relief and a return to a more stable emotional state each month.

Throughout history, the mental health of women has been a complex interplay of misunderstanding, mystification, and marginalization. The journey from ancient beliefs to modern understanding reveals a narrative fraught with gender biases and systemic stigmatization. In ancient times, the mental health of women was often attributed to the so-called wandering womb theory. This concept suggested women's mental and physical health issues were due to a displaced uterus. This archaic belief laid the groundwork for centuries of misdiagnosis and mistreatment, encapsulating women's health issues under the broad and dismissive term *hysteria.* This catch-all diagnosis persisted into the nineteenth century, reflecting a long-standing tradition of medicalizing women's dissent and discomfort, often linking their mental well-being directly to their reproductive functions.

The turn of the twentieth century did little to alleviate these misconceptions. Women's suffrage and the burgeoning feminist movement began to challenge societal norms, yet the medical field continued to pathologize female independence and ambition. Assertions from the era suggested that women stepping beyond their traditional roles were not just unconventional but mentally ill. This period also saw the advent of brutal treatments aimed at curbing women's supposed hysteria, ranging from enforced rest and isolation to more extreme measures like clitoridectomy or oophorectomy, often without consent or informed understanding of the consequences.[123] Such treatments were grounded not in empathy or genuine therapeutic intent but in a desire to control and conform women's behavior to societal expectations.

The late twentieth century marked a significant turning point in the perception and treatment of mental health issues in women, with the feminist movement playing a crucial role in advocating for change. The American Psychological Association's decision in 1980 to replace hysteria with more specific diagnoses like conversion disorder reflected a broader shift toward recognizing the unique mental health challenges faced by women. This period also saw increased attention to the impact of hormonal changes, sexual violence, and societal pressures on women's mental health. Despite these advances, the struggle against stigma and gender-sensitive mental healthcare continues. Today, the conversation is expanding to include the potential of psychedelics in treating conditions uniquely prevalent among women, such as postpartum depression, PMDD, and trauma from sexual violence, signaling a hopeful direction toward more inclusive and effective mental health solutions.

In the realm of mental health, sex plays a critical role, especially in how conditions manifest and affect individuals differently. Among females, depression and anxiety stand out as particularly prevalent, underpinned by a complex interplay of hormonal fluctuations, societal pressures, and unique stressors. Conditions like PMDD, postpartum depression, and perimenopause-related depression underscore the significant impact of reproductive-related hormonal changes on mental well-being. Research has yet to find significant sex differences in the diagnosis rates of schizophrenia and bipolar disorder. However, the symptomatology and course of these illnesses can vary distinctly between females and males.[124] This nuanced understanding of mental health underscores the necessity of sex-specific research and tailored treatment approaches to address the unique challenges females face effectively.

The intersection of mental health and societal factors reveals a distressing picture, particularly in the context of suicide rates among females. The Youth Risk Behaviors Survey highlights a concerning trend, with female students reporting suicide attempts at nearly twice the rate of their male counterparts.[125] This alarming statistic is a stark reminder of the urgent need for targeted mental health interventions and support systems that address the specific needs and experiences of females. Moreover, the National Survey on Drug Use and Health sheds light on the broader spectrum of mental health challenges, with adult females reporting suicide attempts more frequently than males, emphasizing the critical need for comprehensive strategies to prevent mental health crises among females.[126]

Military sexual trauma (MST) represents a particularly harrowing challenge within the armed forces, disproportionately affecting women service members. The Department of Veterans Affairs acknowledges that women in the military face a higher risk of MST, which can lead to a cascade of mental health issues, including depression, PTSD, and substance use disorder. Studies reveal that up to one in three women in the military experience MST, underscoring the pervasive nature of this issue.[127] This distressing reality necessitates a robust response, including accessible support services, preventive measures, and a culture shift within military institutions to protect and support the mental health of all service members, particularly women.

Violence against women, whether through intimate partner violence, workplace harassment, or sexual assault, is a significant driver of mental illness. The profound impact of such trauma on women's mental health cannot be overstated, with survivors facing an increased risk of developing conditions such as depression, anxiety, and PTSD. The statistics are a sobering reminder of the pervasive nature of gender-based violence and its deep-seated effects on mental well-being. As society grapples with these issues, it is imperative to foster a supportive environment that addresses the root causes of violence against women, ensures accessible and compassionate care for survivors, and ultimately, mitigates the mental health fallout of such pervasive societal issues.

The resurgence of interest in psychedelics, once relegated to the fringes of medical research due to decades of stigma and legal prohibitions, heralds a potentially transformative era in the treatment of women's mental health issues. With an increasing number of clinical trials exploring the therapeutic benefits of substances such as ketamine, MDMA, and psilocybin (mushrooms), there's a burgeoning optimism about their efficacy in addressing conditions like depression, PTSD, and the unique psychological challenges faced by women. Notably, the FDA's designation of MDMA and psilocybin as "breakthrough therapies" for PTSD and treatment-resistant depression, respectively, underscores the significant potential these substances hold. Moreover, the Multidisciplinary Association for Psychedelic Studies (MAPS) and the Centre for Psychedelic Research at Imperial College London are pioneering research into the use of MDMA and psilocybin-assisted therapy for eating disorders, a realm where women are disproportionately affected. This shift toward embracing psychedelics as viable treatment options could revolutionize the mental health landscape, offering hope and novel solutions to those who have long struggled with traditional therapies. As we stand on the cusp of this new frontier, it's imperative to navigate the balance between harnessing the profound benefits of psychedelic-assisted therapy and safeguarding against potential misuse, ensuring that this promising avenue for healing is accessible and effectively tailored to the needs of women across the spectrum of mental health challenges.

As we continue to challenge and dismantle the remnants of stigma and gender bias in mental health, the promise of inclusive, effective, and compassionate care becomes a beacon of hope. The path forward requires a continued commitment to research, education, and advocacy, ensuring that the mental healthcare system evolves to meet every woman's needs with the dignity, respect, and efficacy she deserves. FemTech startups and programs are paving this path for improved mental health for every woman.

## Jessica Gaulton, MD, MPH, Founder and CEO at FamilyWell Health

*FamilyWell Health is a digital behavioral health company prioritizing the maternal mental health crisis by integrating obstetric practices with mental health services. Their goal is to provide accessible services for pregnant and postpartum patients. Episode 204 aired April 12, 2023.*

### What is postpartum depression? How prevalent is it? What are current treatments?

Postpartum depression (PPD) is a complex and serious mood disorder that can occur in women after childbirth. It involves physical, emotional, and behavioral changes that can overwhelm new mothers. It's more than just the baby blues, which tends to be milder and resolves itself quickly. PPD can include symptoms such as deep sadness, feelings of emptiness, withdrawal from family and friends, and in more severe cases, thoughts of harming oneself or the baby.

The prevalence of PPD is quite significant and has been increasing, especially in light of recent global challenges like the COVID-19 pandemic. Studies suggest that up to one in three new mothers may experience some form of postpartum depression, which is a substantial increase from the previously estimated one in five.

A holistic and personalized approach is often the most effective in terms of treatment. This can include therapy, such as cognitive behavioral therapy or interpersonal therapy, and medication like antidepressants, depending on the severity of the symptoms. It's important to consider each individual's unique situation, including their medical history, personal preferences, and specific symptoms. In addition, providing strong social support, and educational resources, and creating a nonjudgmental space for new mothers to share their experiences are crucial components of comprehensive care.

Furthermore, integrating mental healthcare into obstetric services is a vital step forward. This means ensuring that ob-gyns have the tools and knowledge to identify and manage PPD, offering services like in-clinic therapists and digital platforms for continuous support. By doing so, we can create a more seamless and supportive healthcare journey for new mothers, ensuring they receive the care they need during this critical period.

**How is FamilyWell helping women with postpartum depression?**

FamilyWell is revolutionizing the way we approach and treat postpartum depression, focusing on accessibility, integration, and personalized care. Our mission is to bridge the significant gaps in mental health services for new mothers, especially those facing postpartum depression.

First, we integrate our services directly into OB-GYN practices, ensuring that mental healthcare is a seamless and standard part of maternal healthcare. This model allows us to catch early signs of postpartum depression and intervene promptly. By embedding trained perinatal mental health therapists in OB-GYN clinics, we make it easier for mothers to receive care in a familiar and trusted setting, breaking down barriers to seeking help.

Additionally, FamilyWell offers a digital platform that includes a range of services such as peer-to-peer text-based coaching, therapy, and psychiatric consultations. Our digital approach expands access, allowing mothers to receive support from the comfort of their homes. This is particularly crucial for new mothers who might find it challenging to attend in-person appointments due to constraints like physical recovery, childcare issues, or transportation challenges.

Our peer-to-peer coaching model is a cornerstone of our approach. It's based on empathy, shared experiences, and emotional support, often missing in traditional healthcare settings. Our coaches, who have navigated their own mental health journeys, offer encouragement and understanding, fostering a community of support that many new mothers desperately need.

Moreover, we're focused on tailoring our services to each mother's unique needs. Recognizing that every mother's experience with postpartum depression is different, we customize our care plans to include a combination of therapy, medication management, and continuous support.

This holistic approach ensures that we address not just the symptoms but also the root causes and individual factors contributing to each mother's condition.

Last, FamilyWell is deeply committed to making mental healthcare equitable and accessible. We work with both Medicaid and commercial insurance providers, emphasizing the need to serve all mothers, regardless of their socioeconomic status. By navigating and advocating within the healthcare system, we aim to make quality mental healthcare a right, not a privilege. Because having access to mental health support should be easy and accessible.

## Kim Palmer, Founder at Clementine

*Clementine developed a hypnotherapy application designed to help women feel calm and confident and get better sleep.*
*Episode 94 aired March 1, 2021.*

### Is women's mental health being addressed adequately?

Women's mental health is currently facing significant challenges, particularly in terms of anxiety and depression. These mental health issues are not only pervasive but are also on the rise, impacting women across various age groups, with younger women aged nineteen to thirty experiencing these concerns more acutely. According to recent studies, such as one from UCL, the gap in stress and anxiety between men and women is widening, exacerbating the situation.

Anxiety and stress, when left unaddressed, can lead to a detrimental cycle affecting sleep patterns, and leading to increased irritability, unhealthy coping mechanisms such as overeating, self-medicating, or excessive drinking, and a decrease in productivity. This cycle, in turn, can severely impact self-esteem and confidence. Self-esteem relates to one's self-worth, while confidence is about belief in one's abilities. The erosion of self-esteem can lead to diminished confidence, influencing women's aspirations, social participation, and, ultimately, their presence in leadership roles and their pursuit of career opportunities.

The societal pressures on women, from appearance to fulfilling specific roles by certain ages, contribute significantly to these mental health challenges. From a young age, women are conditioned to prioritize their appearance over their abilities, with reports indicating that 87 percent of girls aged eleven to twenty-one believe women are judged more on their appearance than their abilities. This skewed perception can lead to poor body image, lower confidence, reduced aspirations, and decreased social participation, perpetuating a cycle that affects women's mental health and their ability to thrive in various aspects of life.

Addressing these issues requires a multifaceted approach, including therapeutic interventions like hypnotherapy, which has been shown to be effective in coping with stress, anxiety, and improving self-esteem and confidence. Hypnotherapy, especially cognitive hypnotherapy, offers a holistic approach by incorporating techniques from cognitive behavioral therapy (CBT), neuro-linguistic programming (NLP), and coaching. It's designed to rewire negative thinking patterns and promote a more positive self-view, providing women with the tools they need to break the cycle of anxiety and stress and improve their mental well-being.

**How does the Clementine app support women's mental health?**

Clementine is a hypnotherapy app designed with women in mind, focusing on those feeling stressed, overwhelmed, anxious, or simply flat. It's like having a coping tool in your pocket to help you calm down, regain confidence, and tackle life with more gusto. What sets Clementine apart is its holistic approach to therapy. We're not just another meditation app but about real, tangible change. By using cognitive hypnotherapy, we blend various techniques like CBT, NLP, and traditional coaching methods to directly address the root causes of stress and anxiety. This combination isn't just about temporary relief; it's about rewiring the brain for long-term resilience and self-esteem.

Clementine uniquely serves women's mental health by recognizing the specific challenges women face today. Whether it's the pressure to perform at work, societal expectations on appearance, or the constant juggling of personal life, Clementine says, "We get it." Our sessions are designed to tackle these unique stressors head-on, providing a toolkit for lasting mental wellness. From helping women start their day right to managing those afternoon slumps and ensuring they get a good night's sleep, Clementine is here to support women through every up and down, making mental healthcare accessible, effective, and, most importantly, tailored to the real experiences of women. It's incredible to see how personalized tools are becoming for various mental health challenges.

## Aneela Idnani, Cofounder at HabitAware

*"Keen" awareness smart bracelet and app puts you in control of nail biting, skin picking, and hairpulling. Episode 37 aired August 17, 2020.*

### What mental health conditions is HabitAware addressing?

Repetitive behavior conditions are known as body-focused repetitive behaviors (BFRBs), encompassing conditions like trichotillomania (hair-pulling), dermatillomania (skin picking), and onychophagia (nail biting). These conditions can affect women differently, often starting in the teen-age years and influenced by hormonal changes. The prevalence of BFRBs is estimated to be around 2 to 5 percent of the US population. Still, it's believed that these conditions are underreported, particularly among women, due to the shame and stigma associated with them.

Women may be more likely to seek help for BFRBs because societal norms and pressures around beauty can make these behaviors particularly distressing for them. For example, hair, skin, and nails are often tied to societal beauty standards for women, making conditions like trichotillomania and dermatillomania more visible and, consequently, more likely to be addressed. Additionally, hormonal fluctuations, such as those during puberty, pregnancy, and menopause, can exacerbate these conditions, suggesting a potential link between hormones and BFRBs.

Despite the apparent gender disparity in BFRBs, there is still much to learn about these conditions, their causes, and their prevalence among different demographics. More research is needed to fully understand BFRBs and develop effective treatments that can address the specific needs of those affected, including the unique challenges women face.

### What product does HabitAware offer? Why did you start this company?

HabitAware is a technology company I cofounded, centered around creating awareness for individuals suffering from BFRBs. We developed Keen, a smart bracelet designed to bring these subconscious behaviors into the conscious realm, enabling users to take control and work toward changing their habits.

Keen uses customized gesture detection technology. Users train the bracelet to recognize the specific gestures associated with their BFRB. When Keen detects the trained gesture, it vibrates, gently notifying the user of the behavior. This moment of awareness allows the individual to choose a different action, breaking the cycle of automatic behavior.

The inspiration for HabitAware came from my personal struggle with trichotillomania, a condition I hid for over twenty years. After a pivotal moment when my husband noticed my hairpulling, we brainstormed a solution that could help me and others facing similar challenges. Our mission with HabitAware is to empower individuals by increasing self-awareness and providing a tool that supports behavior change, ultimately fostering self-healing and improving lives.

## Erin Parks, PhD, Cofounder and CCO at Equip Health

*Equip Health provides a virtual eating disorder treatment program designed to help families recover from eating disorders at home.*
*Episode 164 aired April 17, 2022.*

### How common are eating disorders?

An eating disorder encompasses a range of psychological conditions characterized by abnormal or disturbed eating habits, which can significantly impact one's health, emotions, and ability to function in various areas of life. These disorders include anorexia nervosa, bulimia nervosa, binge eating disorder, and others, affecting millions globally. Current statistics indicate that nearly thirty million Americans will experience an eating disorder at some point in their lives, yet only about 20 percent will receive appropriate treatment. While eating disorders are often viewed through a gendered lens, primarily affecting women, they indiscriminately impact individuals across all genders, ages, ethnicities, and backgrounds. It's a misconception that these disorders solely affect women; men and nonbinary individuals also suffer from eating disorders, albeit often underdiagnosed due to prevailing stereotypes and stigmas. The pandemic has seen a surge in cases, with about a 70 percent increase in eating disorders, highlighting the need for accessible, evidence-based treatment options like those provided by Equip Health. This escalation underscores the profound impact of isolation, heightened emotional distress, and increased exposure to triggering content on social media.

Current treatment options for people with eating disorders vary widely but ideally should be evidence-based and tailored to the individual's specific needs. The mainstay treatments include cognitive behavioral therapy (CBT), which is particularly effective for bulimia nervosa and binge eating disorder. Family-based treatment (FBT) is the gold standard for adolescents with anorexia nervosa, emphasizing the role of the family in the recovery process. There are also specialized forms of therapy, such as dialectical behavior therapy (DBT) and acceptance and commitment therapy (ACT), which can be helpful for addressing the underlying emotional and behavioral issues associated with eating disorders. Medication, such as antidepressants, may be used alongside psychotherapy to treat co-occurring mental health conditions like depression or anxiety. Nutritional counseling and medical monitoring are crucial components of comprehensive care, ensuring physical health is addressed alongside psychological well-being. At Equip Health, we integrate these approaches, providing a multidisciplinary team for each patient to offer a holistic and personalized treatment plan, delivered virtually to increase accessibility and convenience for families.

## What is Equip Health?

Equip Health is a fully virtual treatment provider for eating disorders, aiming to make comprehensive, evidence-based care accessible to those in need. We address eating disorders by providing a five-person treatment team for each patient, which includes a medical provider, a dietitian, a therapist for individual and family therapy, a peer mentor in recovery from an eating disorder, and a family mentor. This multidisciplinary approach ensures comprehensive support, catering to the unique needs of each individual and their family. Our model is designed to treat patients in the comfort of their homes, making recovery a family-centered process.

Despite affecting everyone, eating disorder research receives inadequate funding, with less than $1 per patient in NIH research dollars compared to $75 for the next least-funded mental health disorder. The misrepresentation of eating disorders as a female-centric illness contributes to the lack of funding and accessibility in treatment.

Equip Health's mission extends beyond treatment; we advocate for increased awareness, research, and funding to address the pervasive challenge of eating disorders. Our service is structured to bridge the gap in effective treatment options, emphasizing the importance of early intervention and the role of family and community support in the journey to recovery. There are many mental health conditions that can benefit from additional solutions and tools outside of typical pharmaceutical drugs.

## Juliette McClendon, PhD, Former Director of Medical Affairs at Big Health

*Big Health's mission is to help millions back to good mental health by providing safe and effective non-drug alternatives for the most common mental health conditions including insomnia, anxiety, and depression. Episode 144 aired December 7, 2021.*

### What is insomnia? Does it disproportionately affect women?

Insomnia is a mental health condition characterized by difficulty falling asleep, staying asleep, or obtaining restorative sleep, significantly impacting daily functioning over a prolonged period. It's not just about struggling to sleep for a night or two; it's a chronic issue that can deeply affect one's quality of life. Insomnia is indeed considered a mental health condition because it's closely linked with various psychological processes and stressors that can exacerbate or contribute to the maintenance of sleep problems.

Yes, insomnia does disproportionately affect women. This disparity can be attributed to several factors, including biological, psychological, and social stressors uniquely or more prevalently experienced by women. For instance, hormonal fluctuations associated with menstrual cycles, pregnancy, and menopause can significantly impact sleep quality. Additionally, women often bear a heavier burden of caregiving responsibilities and emotional labor, both within families and as part of the workforce, contributing to higher stress levels and, consequently, sleep disturbances.

The mental health aspect of insomnia underscores the bidirectional relationship between sleep and psychological well-being. Poor sleep can lead to or exacerbate mental health issues such as depression and anxiety. In contrast, these mental health conditions can, in turn, worsen sleep quality, creating a vicious cycle that can be challenging to break. Addressing insomnia from a mental health perspective allows for a more holistic approach to treatment, focusing not only on sleep itself but also on the underlying factors contributing to sleep problems.

### What is a digital therapeutic?

A digital therapeutic is essentially software clinically evaluated to produce measurable health outcomes. It's not just an app or a tool but a sophisticated program that delivers evidence-based therapeutic interventions directly to users. These interventions are based on solid research, including randomized controlled trials, ensuring they are as effective as possible. At Big Health, our digital therapeutics, such as Sleepio for insomnia and Daylight for anxiety, are grounded in cognitive behavioral therapy principles, offering users guided, interactive, and personalized therapy sessions.

Digital therapeutics offer several advantages over psychiatric medication. First, they come with no serious adverse effects, making them a safer option for many individuals. The risk of dependency, withdrawal, or other harmful side effects associated with some psychiatric medications is entirely absent. Second, they're highly accessible and scalable. Since they're software-based, people can access these therapies anytime and anywhere, fitting treatment into their lives without the need to visit a healthcare provider or wait for an appointment. This accessibility can significantly reduce barriers to receiving timely and effective care. Finally, digital therapeutics empower individuals by providing them with tools and skills to manage their conditions actively, promoting long-term resilience and well-being beyond treatment.

* * *

In this chapter on mental health, we explore the profound impact that mental health disorders have on women, underscoring the importance of acknowledging and addressing these issues with compassion and precision. The narrative woven throughout the chapter illustrates not only the pervasive nature of mental health challenges among women but also the societal and physiological complexities that contribute to these conditions. The chapter highlights the critical need for increased awareness, improved healthcare responses, and more substantial support systems to address the mental health needs of women effectively. It calls for a paradigm shift toward a more informed and inclusive approach to mental healthcare that recognizes the specific needs of women, ensuring that they receive the support necessary to lead healthy, fulfilled lives. The emerging use of innovative technologies and therapies offers hope for more effective management and treatment of mental health disorders, promising a future where mental health parity is a reality for all women.

# Chapter 13
# Chronic Conditions

**ALIYAH, A VIBRANT YOUNG PROFESSIONAL,** had been battling a constellation of bewildering symptoms for over a year. She noticed unexplained weight gain, persistent fatigue, and nagging joint pain, accompanied by increasingly irregular menstrual cycles. Despite these concerning changes, Aliyah chalked it up to stress from her demanding job and perhaps a bit of a poor diet. Being generally healthy, she minimized the severity of her symptoms, attributing them to the hustle and bustle of her active lifestyle. Her life continued at its relentless pace, with Aliyah pushing her health concerns to the back of her mind, convinced they were nothing that a little rest couldn't fix.

One evening, while catching up with friends at a local café, Aliyah casually mentioned her frustrating symptoms. Her friend Mia listened intently, then shared that her mother had experienced similar issues and was diagnosed with Hashimoto's—a common yet often overlooked autoimmune disorder affecting the thyroid, especially prevalent among women. Mia explained that women are significantly more likely than men to develop thyroid issues, with about one in eight women facing thyroid dysfunction in their lifetime. This conversation was a turning point for Aliyah; for the first time, she felt that her symptoms might have a tangible explanation. Feeling empowered by this newfound knowledge, Aliyah sought medical advice and requested a blood test to check her thyroid levels, hopeful that she was finally on the path to finding answers and regaining control over her health.

Chronic conditions are conditions or diseases that are persistent or otherwise long-lasting in their effects or diseases that come with time. The term *chronic* is often applied when the course of the disease lasts for more than three months. These conditions range from mental health disorders such as depression and anxiety, to physical illnesses like diabetes, heart disease, and autoimmune diseases. The prevalence of chronic conditions is a growing public health concern, with more than half of US adults having at least one chronic disease.[128] Notably, chronic conditions do not affect all individuals equally; they disproportionately impact women, both in prevalence and severity.[129] This disparity is exacerbated by gender biases in healthcare, leading to underdiagnosis, delayed treatment, and insufficient research focused on women's health issues.[130]

Data from the 2018 National Health Interview Survey (NHIS) estimate more than half (51.8 percent) of adults in the US had at least one of ten commonly diagnosed chronic conditions (arthritis, cancer, chronic obstructive pulmonary disease, coronary heart disease, asthma, diabetes, hepatitis, hypertension, stroke, and renal dysfunction), and 27.2 percent of US adults had multiple chronic conditions.[131] A cross-sectional analysis of the National Health and Nutrition Examination Survey (NHANES) demonstrated 59.6 percent of US civilians twenty years or older had multimorbidity with two or more chronic conditions, 38.5 percent had three or more chronic conditions, and 22.7 percent had more than four chronic conditions.[132]

Statistics reveal that certain chronic conditions, including hypertension, arthritis, depression, and osteoporosis, occur more frequently in women than in men.[133] Data from the Centers for Medicare and Medicaid Services highlight that these conditions are not only more common in women but also contribute to a higher prevalence of multimorbidity among female patients.[134] This gender disparity in chronic disease prevalence underscores the urgent need for a healthcare system that recognizes and addresses the unique challenges faced by women. Despite women making up nearly half of the population, there exists a significant gap in medical research and clinical trials that focuses on conditions predominantly affecting women. A recent evaluation estimated that fewer than a third of published studies reported at least one outcome by sex or explicitly included sex as a covariate in statistical analysis, with explanations for excluding sex in analyses rare.[135] This lack of gender-specific research hinders the development of effective diagnostic tools and treatments tailored to women's health needs.

Chronic conditions affecting women include a wide array of diseases, each with its unique challenges. For instance, autoimmune diseases, which are more prevalent in women, often present with complex symptoms that can be difficult to diagnose and manage.[136] Furthermore, conditions like osteoporosis pose a significant risk to women's health as they age, emphasizing the need for targeted prevention and treatment strategies. The impact of these chronic conditions on women's lives is profound, affecting their physical health, mental well-being, and quality of life. As such, healthcare providers, researchers, and policymakers must prioritize women's health and bridge the gap in research and care for chronic conditions.

Delays in diagnosing women's chronic conditions have become a critical issue, compounded by systemic gender biases in healthcare. A large 2019 population study at the University of Copenhagen demonstrated that men are diagnosed with chronic conditions at comparatively younger ages than women and that women on average waited two to five years longer than men to obtain a diagnosis.[137] In 2019, Westergaard et al. showed that even where there is equal and uniform access to healthcare, there is a marked difference between the diagnosis of diseases affecting men and women.[138] For 770 disease types considered as part of this Danish study, there was an overall gap of four years in diagnosis between women and men.[139]

This delay is not just inconvenient; it can have serious implications for treatment outcomes and overall quality of life. Women suffering from conditions like endometriosis or autoimmune diseases report years of navigating the healthcare system before obtaining a correct diagnosis. This prolonged journey to diagnosis exacerbates their conditions, leading to unnecessary suffering and, in some cases, irreversible damage. The underrepresentation of women in clinical research further compounds this issue, with most of the medical research historically centered on male subjects. This gender disparity in medical research overlooks the biological and physiological differences between the sexes, leading to a healthcare system that is often ill-equipped to address women's specific health needs.

A survey by HealthCentral Corporation revealed that over 10 percent of women, twice the percentage of men, feel uneasy with their healthcare providers, inhibiting them from fully disclosing their symptoms or the ways they are managing their health issues.[140] Furthermore, 15 percent of the female respondents reported a lack of trust in the healthcare system's ability to provide accurate diagnoses and effective treatments, a stark contrast to the mere 6 percent of women who consistently trust the healthcare system, compared to men who are over three times as likely to have trust in their doctor's decisions.[141] The roots of this distrust are multifaceted; notably, around 20 percent of women reported experiencing harm or disrespect from medical professionals, a figure that doubles that of men's experiences.[142] This percentage increases to 26 percent among women aged eighteen to forty-nine.[143] Additionally, over 30 percent of women reported experiencing slow diagnostic processes, a sentiment shared by only 20 percent of men, with more than half of these women attributing the delay to the complexity of their conditions, and 7 percent to gender bias.[144]

The repercussions of diagnostic delays are significant, extending to treatment delays. Alarmingly, 14 percent of women battling chronic conditions reported that their healthcare providers are ineffective at recognizing their symptoms, a rate that is double that of men.[145] Furthermore, dissatisfaction with healthcare providers, their staff, and the location of care is more prevalent among women, with 10 percent expressing outright dissatisfaction, a rate again double that of their male counterparts. Financially, chronic health issues impact women's finances more severely, with 30 percent of women feeling the strain compared to 23 percent of men, as per the HealthCentral Corporation survey.[146] This financial burden is even more pronounced among Black women, who face significant challenges in accessing quality care.

Additionally, obtaining referrals and coverage for psychological counseling proves to be a significant hurdle for nearly a quarter of midlife women, with 20 percent facing difficulties in securing such essential services.[147]

The gender pain gap, a critical aspect of the broader issue, refers to the phenomenon where women's pain is taken less seriously than men's by healthcare professionals. This gap exists due to deeply ingrained gender biases and stereotypes that paint women as overly emotional or prone to exaggeration. Statistics reveal that women are more likely to be prescribed sedatives rather than pain medication, reflecting a troubling trend of dismissing women's pain experiences.[148] Studies, such as "The Girl

Who Cried Pain," highlight that women report more severe and frequent pain compared to men but receive less aggressive treatment.[149] This gap affects the quality of care women receive and diminishes their trust in the healthcare system. The impact of the gender pain gap is far-reaching, affecting not just individual women but society at large, as it contributes to a cycle of underdiagnosis and undertreatment of women's health issues.

Twenty-two percent of females endure severe pain daily, a situation often neglected by the healthcare system, inadequately represented in scientific studies, and minimized due to deep-seated gender biases, leading to a lack of understanding and proper treatment for their pain.[150] The disproportionate incidence of chronic pain among sexes is well-documented, with females experiencing discomfort at a rate 6 percent higher than their male counterparts.[151] This disparity is evident in conditions like back, hip, and knee pain, migraines, arthritis, lupus, fibromyalgia, and uniquely female conditions including endometriosis, interstitial cystitis, vulvodynia, and pelvic girdle syndrome, which specifically affects the area around the pelvic joints and lower back.

According to a survey conducted by HealthyWomen in 2019, nearly half (45 percent) of the participants felt that their pain was not taken seriously by their healthcare providers.[152] This sentiment is supported by data showing that women in pain are more frequently prescribed sedatives rather than pain-relieving medication compared to men. Furthermore, the discrepancy in pain management continues in emergency rooms, where the average wait time for men to receive pain medication for acute abdominal pain is forty-nine minutes. In contrast, women wait approximately sixty-five minutes for the same relief.[153] Additionally, women are less likely than men by half to be administered painkillers following coronary bypass surgery.

The disparity in pain perception and treatment is even more pronounced among Black women. A 2016 study revealed that 50 percent of medical students and residents held at least one of three incorrect beliefs about biological differences between Black and White individuals, such as the sensitivity of nerve endings, thickness of skin, and speed of blood coagulation.[154] According to Dunkley, these misconceptions must be corrected through medical education and training to prevent their continuation.

The consequences of these systemic biases and gaps in care are profound. Women's health conditions are often misdiagnosed or dismissed, leading to delays in receiving necessary care and treatment. For example, conditions like myocardial infarction (heart attack) present differently in women than in men. Yet, the lack of awareness and understanding among healthcare providers means women's symptoms are often overlooked or misinterpreted. This not only puts women's lives at risk but also contributes to a wider gap in health equity. One in three women who seek medical help for a women's health condition are still awaiting a diagnosis, with an average of two years and three months for chronic conditions.[155]

Addressing these disparities demands concerted efforts from healthcare providers, researchers, and policymakers to foster a healthcare environment where gender bias is eradicated, and equitable treatment is not just an ideal but a reality. Bridging this gap benefits women and enriches the entire spectrum of healthcare by ensuring diverse, comprehensive, and effective medical practices that cater to all segments of society. It is a call to action for a more inclusive healthcare system that acknowledges and addresses the specific challenges faced by women with chronic conditions, ensuring that gender no longer dictates the quality of care and treatment received.

## Hormonal Imbalance

### Roya Pakzad, Founder and CEO at Feminade

*Feminade is an online concierge for women's hormone and reproductive health. We help women get to the root cause of their symptoms through advanced at-home testing, telehealth, evidence-based holistic treatments, and education. Episode 8 aired May 4, 2020.*

#### What is hormonal imbalance?

Hormonal imbalance is a pervasive issue affecting a vast majority of women, with symptoms that can significantly impact their quality of life. It occurs when there's a disproportion in the body's levels of hormones like estrogen, progesterone, cortisol, and testosterone, which are crucial for various bodily functions. Hormonal imbalances can lead to a range of symptoms, including but not limited to PMS, depression, low libido, hair loss, cystic acne, and irregular or painful menstrual cycles. It's essential to understand that these symptoms are abnormal and indicate that the body is signaling an underlying issue.

Birth control is often prescribed to manage symptoms of hormonal imbalance. The rationale behind this approach is that birth control pills contain synthetic hormones that can regulate menstrual cycles and alleviate symptoms associated with hormonal imbalances. However, this treatment method doesn't address the root cause of the imbalance. Instead, it can act as a temporary fix, masking the symptoms without solving the underlying problem. Moreover, birth control pills can deplete the body of vital nutrients and vitamins, potentially leading to other health issues.

While birth control can offer a temporary solution for symptom management, it's crucial to approach hormonal imbalance with a more holistic perspective. This includes exploring natural remedies, dietary changes, and lifestyle adjustments that can help restore hormonal balance naturally. For example, magnesium, zinc, selenium, and vitamins E, C, A, and D are supplements that can support hormonal health. Additionally, reducing the intake of dairy products, which may contain synthetic hormones, can help balance hormones.

In essence, addressing hormonal imbalance effectively requires a comprehensive approach that goes beyond just taking birth control. It involves understanding the body's signals, making informed choices about treatment options, and adopting a holistic lifestyle that supports overall hormonal health.

### What is Feminade?

Feminade is an online concierge dedicated to women's hormone and reproductive health, aiming to guide women to the root cause of their hormonal imbalance symptoms as quickly and efficiently as possible. Our approach is rooted in naturopathic, holistic, and integrative medicine. We provide women with an at-home Dutch test, the most sensitive and advanced test for assessing hormones and their metabolites—details not available through standard blood or saliva tests. This comprehensive insight allows a nuanced understanding of a woman's hormonal health, enabling tailored and effective treatment plans.

The inception of Feminade was driven by a personal and observed need for a deeper understanding of women's health issues, particularly the widespread dismissal of women's symptoms within the healthcare system. It's alarming that a significant percentage of women experience hormonal imbalance symptoms, yet face a long, often frustrating journey toward diagnosis and effective treatment. The conventional medical practice of prescribing birth control as a blanket solution—without addressing the underlying causes—compelled me to seek a more informed, empowering approach for women. This involves identifying hormonal imbalances through advanced testing and providing education, support, and personalized care through consultations with licensed naturopathic doctors. We look forward to updating our tests and services as more research and models are created to understand women's hormones.

## Caralynn Nowinski Collens, MD, CEO at Dimension Inx

*Dimension Inx is a next-generation biomaterial and biofabrication company developing 3D-printed therapeutic products that direct cells to rebuild healthy tissues. Episode 176 aired August 15, 2022.*

### What is Dimension Inx? What are you building?

Dimension Inx is a regenerative medicine company at the forefront of developing 3D-printed therapeutic products. Our mission revolves around directing cells to rebuild healthy tissue. By leveraging next-generation biomaterials and biofabrication technology, we're creating environments that instruct cells on how to behave properly to regenerate tissue.

Our focus is on products for various therapeutic applications, ranging from bone regeneration to fertility preservation. For instance, our initial product aims at facial reconstruction, where we use our technology to create implants that can regenerate bone, restoring its function. This application is just the beginning.

One of the more innovative products in our pipeline is what we've termed an artificial ovary or a bio-prosthetic ovary. The goal is to replicate the natural ovarian environment as closely as possible, directing oocytes to mature into viable eggs. This project is particularly exciting as it not only represents a significant advancement in fertility preservation but also opens the door to hormone restoration therapies, thereby addressing a wider range of women's health issues. Our approach is deeply rooted in understanding and engineering the microenvironment of cells to optimize their behavior for therapeutic outcomes.

### How could an artificial ovary support hormone imbalance?

An artificial ovary could significantly impact hormone replacement and imbalances by creating a microenvironment that mimics the natural ovarian structure, thus supporting the maturation of follicles into viable eggs without the need for hormone stimulation. This approach leverages advanced manufacturing technologies and a deep understanding of ovarian biology to engineer a system that can function outside the body (ex vivo) for fertility purposes or potentially can be implanted to restore hormone function.

In the case of fertility preservation, the goal is to develop a system where follicles can mature into eggs in a laboratory setting, and then be implanted back into the body for a viable pregnancy, offering a new avenue for IVF without the extensive hormone treatments currently required. For hormone replacement, envisioning a future where these engineered microenvironments could be implanted to restore natural hormone production, addressing conditions like menopause or hormone imbalances caused by ovarian reserve depletion, is within reach.

The challenge lies in replicating the ovary's complex and dynamic environment, which involves not only the biochemical signals but also the mechanical cues that follicles experience during maturation. By creating a synthetic yet biologically familiar environment, cells can be directed to behave in desired ways, such as developing and maturing oocytes or producing essential hormones, thus offering a multifaceted approach to tackling a range of reproductive health issues.

This endeavor taps into the broader field of regenerative medicine, aiming to restore function rather than merely replicate anatomical structures. It represents a convergence of biology, material science, and advanced manufacturing techniques, illustrating a significant shift toward more natural and personalized healthcare solutions. In the future, women can test and monitor their hormones daily and conveniently in their homes.

## Marina Pavlovic Rivas, Cofounder and CEO at Eli Health

*Eli Health enables women to take control of their health across their lives, by providing them with powerful information on their daily hormone profile. Episode 125 aired July 18, 2021.*

## What is Eli Health?

Eli Health is developing a device that measures hormone levels in saliva and interprets those levels to provide insights into various aspects of women's health. The inspiration for Eli Health came from a personal journey, realizing the limited options at the intersection of hormone-free, noninvasive, and effective birth control. However, the vision quickly expanded beyond fertility and contraception to encompass a broader mission. Hormones are crucial in numerous conditions and transitions women experience throughout their lives. By placing hormonal data into women's hands, Eli Health aims to empower them with better control over their health across all stages of life.

The technology we're building enables high-frequency hormone testing over long periods, something not currently available on the market. We're starting with estradiol and progesterone to detect the entire fertile window. Still, our technology allows for expansion to other hormones, supporting a broader range of health insights beyond reproductive health. This encompasses general health, recognizing that many conditions, not specifically exclusive to women but affecting them differently or disproportionately, are driven by hormonal fluctuations.

Our device involves a cartridge with a small sponge placed on the tongue for a few seconds. This cartridge is then inserted into a palm-sized device at home, with results sent to a smartphone within a few minutes. This process is designed to be as easy as brushing your teeth, addressing the need for a hormone monitoring product suited for long-term, everyday use across a woman's life.

Eli Health aims to be present in every home, offering insights at every stage of a woman's life. This will involve further technological development, clinical studies, and research to support additional use cases. We are not just a reproductive health company but a general health company, aiming to address the wide range of conditions influenced by hormonal fluctuations, including those not specific to women but which impact them in unique ways.

## What does the future of hormone testing look like?

Eli Health is pioneering a device for daily saliva hormone measurement, recognizing hormones' profound impact on various aspects of women's health beyond fertility and contraception. By monitoring hormones like estradiol and progesterone, women gain insights into their fertile window with potential applications spanning contraception to broader health concerns. Hormones, central to conditions and transitions experienced by women, when tracked, can empower them with control over their health throughout their lives.

Daily hormone monitoring can reveal fluctuations linked to numerous conditions affecting women, such as migraines or PMS, highlighting the need for a deeper understanding of hormonal impacts. Our technology aims for seamless integration into daily routines, ensuring long-term, high-frequency testing to support health decisions at every life stage. The future of hormone testing promises expansion to additional hormones, addressing a wider range of health insights. Through continuous research and development, Eli Health envisions a world where every woman can access personalized hormonal data, fostering a profound shift toward proactive and informed health management. There are many hormonal conditions women have like PCOS that could greatly benefit from daily hormone testing to better understand and manage their symptoms.

## Megan M. Stewart, Founder and Executive Director at PCOS Awareness Association (PCOSAA)

*PCOS Awareness Association is a nonprofit organization dedicated to the advocacy of polycystic ovarian syndrome or PCOS. The organization and its volunteers are dedicated to raising awareness of this disorder worldwide, providing educational and support services to help people understand what it is and how it can be treated.*
*Episode 127 aired August 2, 2021.*

### What is PCOS Awareness Association?

PCOS Awareness Association, which I founded, provides advocacy, research, resources, support, and information to address the needs of individuals affected by polycystic ovary syndrome (PCOS). I started it due to my personal struggles with PCOS and cervical cancer, realizing the lack of information and support for PCOS. Symptoms began at age nine, but it wasn't until I was sixteen that I received a formal diagnosis. The journey to diagnosis was challenging, involving numerous doctors and specialists, underscoring the need for greater awareness and resources.

PCOS is a prevalent condition, affecting one in five women globally, with over half of them undiagnosed. Our association aims to fill the information gap, offering resources like low-income clinic partnerships for healthcare access, medication discounts, and mental health support through our collaboration with Crisis Text Line. We're also developing educational courses for PCOS patients and medical providers, recognizing the need for more comprehensive education within the medical community.

The future goals of our organization include expanding our reach and resources to aid more individuals, supporting research to uncover the origins and effective treatments for PCOS, and creating programs that address the needs of younger individuals affected by this condition. Through these efforts, PCOS Awareness Association seeks to empower those with PCOS with knowledge, support, and a community, advocating for better healthcare solutions and awareness.

## Why is PCOS underdiagnosed? What is the role of mental health in PCOS?

PCOS is a common hormonal disorder among women of reproductive age, characterized by a variety of symptoms that can affect the body both physically and metabolically. The condition is named for the appearance of multiple small cysts on the ovaries, as seen during an ultrasound, although not all women with PCOS have these cysts. PCOS is also associated with an increased risk of developing health issues like insulin resistance, type 2 diabetes, high cholesterol, high blood pressure, and heart disease. The exact cause of PCOS is unknown, but factors such as genetics, insulin resistance, and higher levels of androgens (male hormones) play significant roles. Managing PCOS typically involves lifestyle changes like diet and exercise, medications to manage symptoms, and treatment of infertility if pregnancy is desired.

PCOS is underdiagnosed primarily due to a lack of awareness and understanding among both individuals and healthcare providers. Many symptoms of PCOS, such as irregular periods, weight gain, and acne, can be mistakenly attributed to other causes or dismissed as normal adolescent changes. This, combined with the variability of symptoms among those affected, complicates diagnosis. Additionally, there's a significant gap in medical education regarding PCOS, often reducing it to a paragraph in medical textbooks, which does not equip healthcare providers with the knowledge to recognize and diagnose it effectively.

Mental health challenges are a critical concern for those with PCOS, stemming from both the physiological impacts of the syndrome and the emotional toll of dealing with a chronic, misunderstood condition. Hormonal imbalances associated with PCOS can directly influence mood, contributing to anxiety and depression. Furthermore, visible symptoms like hair loss, weight gain, and acne can severely affect self-esteem and body image, leading to social withdrawal and heightened stress. The frustration of navigating a healthcare system that lacks a deep understanding of PCOS exacerbates these mental health challenges, often leaving individuals feeling isolated and unsupported. This is why initiatives like Crisis Text Line collaboration are vital, providing immediate mental health support to those struggling with PCOS-related distress.

## Autoimmune

## Rory Stanton, Founder and CEO at Aila Health

*Aila is on a mission to improve the healthcare experience for autoimmune patients, who are disproportionately female. They use data to bring the "invisible" into view, support shared decision-making with a care team, and develop a personalized care plan that works for the patient's life. Episode 129 aired August 16, 2021.*

### What is an autoimmune disease? How common are they?

Autoimmune diseases are conditions in which the immune system mistakenly attacks the body's own tissues, leading to various symptoms and complications. These diseases are remarkably common, with one in six Americans grappling with an autoimmune condition. This is especially true among women, with about 75 percent of autoimmune disease cases occurring in females. The reasons behind this disparity are not fully understood, but hypotheses include hormonal, genetic, and environmental factors.

Stress plays a significant role in exacerbating the symptoms of autoimmune diseases. Many patients report flare-ups or worsening symptoms during periods of stress. Stress can trigger inflammatory responses in the body, which may amplify the symptoms of autoimmune conditions. Managing stress through lifestyle modifications, mindfulness, and other stress reduction techniques can be crucial in managing autoimmune diseases.

**What is Aila and why did you start it?**

The Aila app is a virtual care platform designed for individuals with long-term, complex, chronic illnesses, focusing specifically on autoimmune diseases. It provides users personalized care through data and technology, helping them better manage their conditions. Aila is unique because it aims to deliver a holistic care model, integrating various aspects of health management, including lifestyle modifications, stress management, and nutritional guidance, all tailored to the individual's specific needs and symptoms. We started Aila to address the fragmented care journey many patients with chronic autoimmune conditions face. The inspiration came from seeing friends and family struggle with the diagnostic odyssey and realizing the need for more personalized, accessible care solutions that consider each patient's unique experiences. Our goal is to empower patients with the tools and resources to better manage their health and improve their quality of life.

## Pain

### Abigail Hirsch, PhD, Cofounder and Chief Clinical Officer at Lin Health

*The company's platform provides digital pain care programs that manage patients and connect them to a remote care system. By leveraging telehealth services and nonopioid treatments, the company enables patients to address their unmet needs in the treatment of chronic pain.*
*Episode 145 aired December 7, 2021.*

**Tell us about chronic pain.**

Chronic pain is a disorder that affects approximately one in five Americans, with emerging data suggesting the number could be as high as one in two. It's distinct from acute pain, which is temporary and typically resolves as the body heals, usually within a few months. Chronic pain, however, persists beyond the expected period of healing, lasting more than six months, and significantly disrupts daily living. It's not merely a prolonged version of acute pain. Still, it is considered a health condition in its own right, with the International Classification of Diseases (ICD) recognizing it in its latest revision (ICD-11). This classification shift is crucial as it acknowledges chronic pain's complex nature, where the pain *system* becomes the problem, rather than merely signaling an underlying issue.

Types of chronic pain include primary and secondary pain. Primary pain stands out because it's mostly driven by nervous system dysfunction rather than direct tissue damage, encompassing conditions like fibromyalgia, irritable bowel syndrome, and chronic pelvic pain. Secondary pain is linked directly to another condition, such as arthritis or cancer.

Chronic pain is a reality for one in five Americans and women are disproportionately affected, with conditions like fibromyalgia being significantly more common among women. This disparity may be due to biological, psychological, and social factors, including differences in pain perception, hormonal influences, and potentially gender bias in pain assessment and treatment. The reality that chronic pain conditions, particularly those affecting women, are under-recognized and undertreated in healthcare highlights the need for greater awareness and targeted interventions.

Chronic pain significantly impacts every facet of a woman's life, manifesting as a physical sensation and a comprehensive challenge affecting emotional well-being, social relationships, and professional life. Women experiencing chronic pain often find their daily activities and routines disrupted. The persistent and sometimes unpredictable nature of pain can lead to increased stress, anxiety, and depression, as the struggle to manage symptoms and maintain normalcy becomes overwhelming.

Socially, chronic pain can lead to isolation as women might withdraw from activities and relationships that were once enjoyable but now exacerbate their pain. This isolation can further compound feelings of loneliness and misunderstanding, as others might not fully appreciate the invisible nature of their condition.

Professionally, chronic pain poses significant challenges. It can affect a woman's ability to work, leading to decreased productivity, missed opportunities, and even job loss. The constant battle with pain requires significant energy and focus, which can detract from career aspirations and achievements.

Moreover, the healthcare journey for women with chronic pain is often fraught with additional challenges, including being dismissed or not taken seriously by medical professionals. This can delay accurate diagnosis and effective treatment, exacerbating the sense of frustration and helplessness.

### How is chronic pain treated? How does Lin Health work?

Treatments for chronic pain vary widely, but we're pioneering a digital-first, brain-based approach tailored to each individual's needs at Lin Health. Chronic pain often persists due to a dysfunction in how the brain processes pain signals, rather than ongoing tissue damage. Recognizing this, we focus on retraining the brain's response to pain through techniques grounded in the latest pain science.

Lin Health is a virtual care platform for individuals experiencing chronic pain. We provide a comprehensive, personalized program that combines the expertise of pain specialists with the convenience of digital access. Our approach is rooted in understanding that chronic pain is a complex condition that affects every aspect of a person's life. Therefore, our treatment plans are not one-size-fits-all but are customized to address the multifaceted nature of pain.

We employ innovative methods to help our members manage and alleviate their chronic pain. One key technique is pain reprocessing therapy (PRT), which helps individuals understand the nature of their pain and learn new ways to respond to it. This method is complemented by cognitive behavioral strategies, mindfulness practices, and education about pain science, all aimed at reducing pain sensitivity and improving quality of life. Additionally, we support our members in making lifestyle adjustments that can positively impact their pain experience, such as improving sleep, nutrition, and physical activity.

Our holistic, brain-first approach to pain management sets Lin Health apart. We recognize that chronic pain is not just a physical condition but a complex interplay of biological, psychological, and social factors. By addressing pain from this comprehensive perspective and leveraging the power of digital technology, we can support our members in navigating their pain journey and moving toward a more pain-free life.

* * *

In exploring chronic conditions affecting women, we've uncovered a stark reality. These conditions not only persist with a high degree of prevalence but also carry profound implications due to systemic disparities in diagnosis and treatment. Chronic illnesses such as heart disease, diabetes, and autoimmune disorders disproportionately affect women, presenting unique challenges that are often exacerbated by a healthcare system riddled with gender biases. These biases contribute to delayed diagnoses and inadequate treatment, particularly in conditions predominantly affecting women. Moreover, the intersectionality of these chronic conditions with mental health cannot be overstated, as psychological components often complicate the clinical presentations and outcomes of these diseases. As we navigate this complex landscape, medical research and healthcare policies must pivot toward a more inclusive approach that acknowledges and addresses the specific needs of women. This will ensure that women's health is not only reactive to symptoms but proactive in preventing and managing chronic conditions effectively, ultimately enhancing the quality of life for millions of women.

# Chapter 14
# Beyond Bikini Medicine

**WOMEN'S HEALTH EXTENDS FAR BEYOND** the traditionally emphasized areas of reproductive and breast health, often dubbed "bikini medicine." Increasingly, the medical community recognizes the critical need to research and understand health issues affecting women's brains, bones, hearts, gastrointestinal systems, and blood—areas where gender disparities in research and understanding have profound implications.

In the landscape of neuroscience, a stark contrariety unfolds between the research dedicated to men's and women's brain health, revealing a gender gap that cannot be ignored. Despite women being disproportionately affected by brain-related conditions such as Alzheimer's disease and depression, less than 0.5 percent of neuroscience studies have focused on women's brain health specifically.[156]

This neglect is particularly alarming given the profound influence of sex hormones on neurological functions and the marked differences in disease prevalence. For instance, Alzheimer's disease, a condition that gravely impairs memory and cognitive functions, afflicts women at twice the rate of men, a statistic that remains significant even when accounting for women's longer life expectancy.[157] This gender discrepancy in brain health research not only highlights a critical gap in our scientific understanding but also indicates an urgent need for a more inclusive research agenda that addresses women's unique neurological needs.

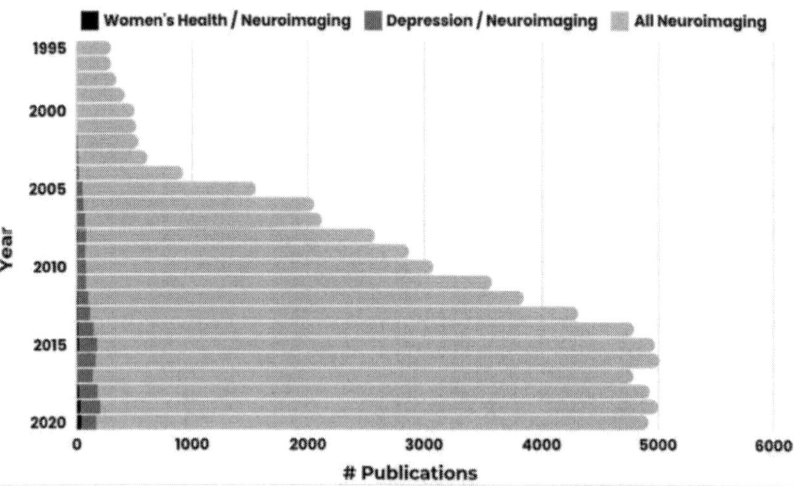


*Figure 13: Women's health factors are severely understudied in neuroimaging research. A historical survey of neuroimaging papers published since 1995 shows the remarkable growth in neuroimaging studies of the human brain. There is a clear disparity for the number of publications that consider aspects of brain health specific to women including menopause, pregnancy, contraceptive use, the menstrual cycle and more, accounting for just 286 out of ~43,000 total publications. Neuroimaging papers published on depression shown for comparison.*[158]

The impact of this research imbalance is far-reaching, affecting the development of targeted treatments and interventions for women. Neurological studies, historically gender-neutral in approach, have often overlooked the nuanced ways in which conditions manifest and progress differently in women. For example, white matter hyperintensities (brain lesions linked to cognitive decline and stroke risk) have been shown to evolve differently in men and women. Monique Breteler, MD, PhD, of the German Center of Neurodegenerative Diseases in Bonn, and coauthors found these brain lesions increase more rapidly in postmenopausal women than in men of a similar age, suggesting hormonal changes plus sex-specific variations in the aging process are defining factors of brain health.[159] This evidence calls for a tailored approach to women's brain health, emphasizing the importance of considering sex as a critical factor in both research and treatment protocols. Without a concerted effort to bridge this gap, women will continue to face a healthcare landscape that is ill-equipped to meet their specific health needs.

The narrative around women's health is undergoing a crucial evolution, extending its focus beyond reproductive health to address the systemic neglect in research and care for conditions like osteoporosis—with women making up 80 percent of the population affected by this bone-weakening disease.[160, 161] Osteoporosis is responsible for more than two million broken bones annually in the United States alone, posing a significant economic burden, with costs projected to reach $25.3 billion (about $78 per person in the US) by 2025.[162] This alarming figure spotlights not just a health crisis but an economic one.

The stark reality is that a woman's risk of experiencing a bone fracture due to osteoporosis is greater than her risk of breast, ovarian, and uterine cancers combined.[163] Yet, the focus on women's bone health remains insufficient in the broader medical discourse, leading to missed opportunities for prevention, early detection, and effective management.

The economic impact of osteoporosis-related fractures extends beyond healthcare costs to include the lost wages and productivity of women forced out of the workforce due to their condition or caregiving responsibilities for family members with similar health issues. Women, often the primary caregivers, face a double burden—managing their health and the health of loved ones—leading to significant financial and emotional strain. Moreover, the ripple effects of such fractures on women's health are profound, with studies showing that one in two women over the age of fifty will experience an osteoporosis-related fracture, compared to just one in four men.[164]

In addition, women over fifty who experience hip fractures are at a greater risk of mortality within the subsequent year compared to those without fractures.[165] This grim reality is a clarion call for targeted interventions to bolster women's bone health, enhance economic productivity, and improve overall well-being.

Addressing this inequality requires a multifaceted approach, beginning with increased investment in bone health research that prioritizes understanding women's unique physiology and the role of menopause and aging in bone density loss (estrogen is needed to protect bone health and density, and this hormone decreases sharply as women reach menopause). There's also a pressing need for widespread public health campaigns that educate women on risk factors and preventive measures, coupled with policy reforms that ensure better access to screening and treatment. Empowering women with the knowledge and resources to take charge of their bone health can lead to earlier detection of osteoporosis, reducing the incidence of fractures and their associated economic and health costs. By spotlighting this overlooked aspect of women's health, we can forge a path toward a future where bone health is recognized as a critical component of women's well-being and economic independence.

In the realm of cardiovascular health, a significant sex disparity persists, rooted in the long-standing medical paradigm that prioritizes male heart health as the standard. This one-size-fits-all approach overlooks critical physiological differences between men and women, leading to underdiagnosis and undertreatment of heart disease in women. Heart disease remains the leading cause of death for women worldwide, with over 60 million women in the United States living with the condition.[166] Yet, awareness among women about their heart disease risk is alarmingly low, with only about half recognizing it as their greatest health threat. This lack of awareness, combined with a healthcare system calibrated to male norms, significantly impacts women's health outcomes.

Research reveals that heart disease manifests differently in women, including distinct symptoms, risk factors, and disease progression. Women are more likely to experience nontraditional symptoms such as nausea, dizziness, and fatigue, which can be easily dismissed or misdiagnosed. Moreover, conditions like preeclampsia and gestational diabetes during pregnancy are now recognized as powerful indicators of future cardiovascular risk. Yet, these female-specific risk factors are often overlooked in traditional heart disease models. Additionally, the prevalence of heart disease in women is influenced by hormonal changes, particularly after menopause. Yet, the impact of these changes is not fully incorporated into current diagnostic and treatment protocols.

High blood pressure is a major risk factor for heart disease but is often underdiagnosed in women. More than fifty-eight million women in the US have high blood pressure or are on medication for the condition, with just 23 percent managing to keep it under control.[167] Black women are nearly 60 percent more likely to have high blood pressure than White women; this highlights the importance of personalized health-risk scores.[168]

The continued reliance on a male-centric paradigm in heart health research and care delivery has real-world consequences for females, from delayed diagnosis to less effective treatments. A 2016 study from Brigham's

Cardiovascular Disease and Pregnancy Program demonstrated that women aged forty or younger with endometriosis were three times more likely to develop heart attack or chest pain, or require treatment for blocked arteries versus peers without endometriosis.[169] For example, the discrepancy in how heart attacks are diagnosed illustrates this issue. Men typically present with chest pain, leading to immediate and aggressive intervention, whereas women's symptoms can be more subtle and are less likely to be immediately attributed to heart conditions. By tailoring diagnostic tools, treatments, and preventive strategies to the specific needs of women, the medical community can close this gap, ensuring better outcomes for women's heart health.

In an increasingly aging society, women bear the brunt of caregiving responsibilities, a role that extends far beyond the confines of love and duty into a realm of significant financial, emotional, and physical tolls.

Women constitute 81 percent of caregivers. This informal caregiving is valued between $148 billion and $188 billion annually. This showcases women's indispensable role in the healthcare ecosystem.[170, 171] Yet, this substantial contribution is unpaid and comes with high costs. Women caregivers navigate this demanding path often at the expense of their careers, personal health, and financial security. Studies reveal that women caregivers may spend as much as 50 percent more time providing care than their male counterparts, spending an average of twelve years out of the workforce raising children or caring for an elderly relative or friend.[172] Even in heterosexual relationships where both partners are working full-time, the woman will take on 40 percent additional caring responsibilities, further exacerbating gender disparities in income, career advancement, and retirement savings.[173]

The caregiver burden also has profound implications for women's mental and physical health. Engaging in long-term caregiving can lead to increased stress, depression, and physical health problems. Caregivers also report higher incidences of chronic conditions such as hypertension and heart disease.[174]

The emotional and physical strain of caregiving is compounded by the financial insecurity often accompanying the role. Women caregivers are more likely to experience job disruptions, a 41 percent reduction of paid working hours, or even early retirement, leading to an estimated $324,044 loss in wages and Social Security benefits over a lifetime.[175] The situation is dire for those caring for individuals with severe health issues like Alzheimer's or stroke, where the caregiving demands are not just more intense but also longer in duration. A longitudinal study published in 2002 found that women who provided at least thirty-six hours of care to a disabled spouse were almost six times more likely than non-caregivers to experience depressive or anxious symptoms.[176] Addressing women caregivers' challenges requires societal acknowledgment of their invaluable contribution and the implementation of supportive policies and resources to mitigate their burdens.

As we navigate through the myriad of health challenges unique to women, from the intricacies of brain and heart conditions to the silent epidemic of osteoporosis and the pervasive issue of gastrointestinal disorders, it becomes abundantly clear that the approach to women's health requires a paradigm shift. The disparities in research, diagnosis, and treatment not only highlight a significant gap in our healthcare system but also call for an urgent reevaluation of how women's health issues are prioritized and addressed. Moreover, the substantial burden placed on women as primary caregivers further exacerbates these health disparities, creating a cycle of stress and illness that impacts not only the individual but also the broader societal fabric. Addressing these issues demands a concerted effort from medical researchers, healthcare providers, policymakers, and society to ensure that women receive comprehensive, nuanced care that considers the full spectrum of their health needs. We hope to build a more equitable and effective healthcare system for all through a collective commitment to understanding and addressing the unique challenges of women's health.

## Brain

### Mary Angela O'Neal, MD, Chief of General Neurology at Brigham and Women's Hospital

*Dr. Mary O'Neal is a renowned expert in women's neurology, currently serving as the director of the Women's Neurology Program at the Brigham and Women's Hospital, a prestigious Harvard Medical School teaching hospital. Episode 189 aired November 28, 2022.*

## What is eclampsia?

Preeclampsia and eclampsia are related pregnancy complications that are both serious and warrant close medical attention. Preeclampsia is a condition characterized by high blood pressure. It typically occurs after the twentieth week of pregnancy and can affect various organ systems, including the liver and kidneys. The exact cause of preeclampsia is not entirely understood, but it's believed to involve several factors, including blood vessel problems, immune system issues, and genetics.

Eclampsia is a more severe progression of preeclampsia and is characterized by the onset of seizures in a woman with preeclampsia. These seizures can be life-threatening for both the mother and the baby. Eclampsia is a medical emergency and requires immediate treatment.

Both conditions can have significant implications for the health of the mother and the baby. They can lead to complications like preterm birth or low birth weight, and in severe cases, can be life-threatening. The only definitive treatment for preeclampsia and eclampsia is the delivery of the baby, which can be challenging if the pregnancy is far from full term. Therefore, management often involves carefully balancing the mother's health and the fetus's development, with close monitoring and, in some cases, early delivery if the situation warrants.

Pregnant women must attend regular prenatal appointments to monitor their blood pressure and other vital signs to catch any signs of preeclampsia early. If diagnosed, management strategies may include medications to control blood pressure, bed rest, and close monitoring until it's safe to deliver the baby.

## How do women's brains change throughout their life?

Women's brains undergo several significant changes throughout their lives, influenced by biological and hormonal factors. These changes start at the fetal stage and continue through old age.

Fetal Development and Childhood: Even in utero, the female brain develops differently from the male brain, influenced by genetic and hormonal factors. These differences continue to evolve during childhood, impacting various aspects of cognitive and emotional development.

Adolescence: The onset of puberty brings about a surge in hormones, notably estrogen, which has a profound impact on the brain. This period is marked by further development and refinement of brain structures and functions, influencing emotional processing, cognitive abilities, and the risk of developing certain neurological or psychiatric conditions.

Reproductive Years: The menstrual cycle can influence brain chemistry and function during a woman's reproductive years. Fluctuations in hormones like estrogen and progesterone can affect mood, cognition, and susceptibility to certain neurological conditions, such as migraines. Additionally, the use of hormonal contraceptives can also have an impact on brain function and structure.

Pregnancy and Postpartum: Pregnancy brings significant hormonal changes that can affect the brain. For instance, some areas of the brain involved in social cognition and emotional regulation may undergo remodeling, potentially enhancing maternal attachment to the newborn. Postpartum women may experience shifts in mood and cognition, partly influenced by rapid hormonal changes after childbirth.

Menopause: As women approach menopause, the decline in estrogen levels can have notable effects on the brain. This can manifest as changes in mood, memory, and cognitive function. Some women may experience increased susceptibility to mood disorders or cognitive decline during this period.

Aging: In later life, women may experience aging-related brain changes. Research suggests that women may have a higher risk of certain age-related neurological conditions, such as Alzheimer's disease, possibly linked to postmenopausal hormonal changes.

Throughout these stages, lifestyle factors, genetics, and environmental influences also play a crucial role in shaping brain health and function. Understanding these changes is vital for developing gender-specific approaches to brain health and disease prevention.

Neurological conditions can take many forms including migraines and headaches.

## Jillian Levovitz, MBA, Former Cofounder and CEO at OcciGuide

*OcciGuide is a revolutionary device that enables clinicians to provide specialized headache relief for many types of headaches, including migraines and post-traumatic headaches. Episode 184 aired October 24, 2022.*

## What are headaches, and how do they affect women?

Headaches are common neurological disorders characterized by head, scalp, or neck pain. They can vary in intensity, duration, and frequency, and are often categorized into different types, including tension headaches, migraines, cluster headaches, and others. Headaches can significantly affect daily life, impairing the ability to work, socialize, and perform everyday tasks.

Women are particularly affected by headaches, especially migraines. Research shows that women are twice as likely as men to experience migraines, which could be linked to hormonal fluctuations. These hormonal changes, particularly those associated with the menstrual cycle, pregnancy, and menopause, can trigger or exacerbate headache episodes in many women.

The impact of headaches on women is multifaceted. It's not just about the physical pain; it also encompasses the psychological and social aspects. Women with frequent headaches may experience increased stress, anxiety, and depression. They might also face challenges in managing their professional and personal responsibilities, affecting their quality of life and overall well-being.

One of the major challenges in understanding and treating headaches in women is the need for more comprehensive research exploring the connection between female hormonal cycles and headache patterns. More studies are needed to fully understand these dynamics, which could lead to better, more personalized treatment strategies for women.

## What is OcciGuide?

OcciGuide is a medical device that offers a novel, nonpharmacological approach to headache treatment. It's a groundbreaking tool that provides a precise, guided method for performing nerve blocks, specifically the occipital nerve block, a well-established procedure for headache relief.

The device is designed to be placed on the back of the head, aligning with key anatomical landmarks. Through this alignment, it accurately locates the occipital nerves. Once these nerves are located, a healthcare provider can inject a local anesthetic like lidocaine into the nerve areas. This injection effectively turns off the pain signals these nerves transmit, relieving headache symptoms.

OcciGuide is particularly beneficial for women suffering from headaches for several reasons. Traditional headache treatments, especially medications, can have various side effects and sometimes are not recommended for women, particularly those who are pregnant or planning to become pregnant. Moreover, OcciGuide's approach to headache relief is fast-acting and can have lasting effects. Women who experience frequent or chronic headaches can find significant relief without the need for continuous medication use, which can be a game-changer in terms of quality of life and overall health. The device provides a nonhormonal treatment option, especially relevant for women who experience headaches related to hormonal fluctuations.

The brain is an incredibly complex organ that affects every aspect of life. This includes how the brain functions and processes manifesting in different neurodivergence.

## Jenny Wu, Copresident and Chief Product Officer at Understood

*Understood is a nonprofit dedicated to shaping the world for difference. We provide resources and support so people who learn and think differently can thrive in school, at work, and throughout life.*
*Episode 183 aired October 3, 2022.*

### How are neurological conditions like ADHD different in females and males?

ADHD manifests differently in females and males, primarily due to biological, psychological, and social factors. Traditionally, ADHD has been perceived as a condition more prevalent in males, mainly because of its more noticeable symptoms like hyperactivity and impulsiveness, which are more commonly observed in boys. However, this doesn't mean that ADHD affects males more frequently than females; rather, it's often underdiagnosed in females.

In females, ADHD symptoms can be more subtle and internalized compared to males. Girls and women with ADHD may experience inattentiveness, daydreaming, and disorganization, which can be easily overlooked or misattributed to other causes. Unfortunately, this often leads to a delayed diagnosis in females, which can have significant impacts on their self-esteem, academic performance, and overall mental health.

Moreover, societal expectations and gender roles play a part. Girls are often encouraged to be quieter and more compliant, which can mask hyperactive or impulsive behaviors that are more readily identified in boys. This societal bias contributes to the underdiagnosis or misdiagnosis of ADHD in females.

Additionally, hormonal fluctuations in females can influence ADHD symptoms. Research indicates that hormonal changes during menstruation, pregnancy, and menopause can affect the severity and presentation of ADHD symptoms in women. Understanding this gender-specific aspect of ADHD is crucial for effective management and treatment.

Overall, the differences in how ADHD presents in females and males highlight the need for greater awareness and more gender-sensitive diagnostic criteria. Healthcare professionals, educators, and parents need to recognize these differences to ensure that females with ADHD receive appropriate support and treatment.

## Karyn Frick, PhD, Cofounder and Chief Scientific Officer at Estrigenix

*Estrigenix is dedicated to developing safe medications that target the side effects of menopause, such as hot flashes and memory impairments, without the adverse side effects associated with traditional estrogen therapies. Episode 208 aired May 10, 2023.*

### What is the role of estrogen in the brain?

Estrogen plays a crucial role in the brain beyond its traditional association with reproduction. It's a critical hormone significantly impacting cognitive functions, including memory and mood. Estrogen interacts with specific receptors in the brain, acting as a messenger delivering vital instructions to brain cells. These instructions can range from gene expression changes to rapid molecular alterations affecting neuronal communication.

My research has focused on understanding the specific cellular and molecular mechanisms through which estrogens influence memory. We've discovered that estrogen receptors are abundant in critical areas of the brain, such as the hippocampus and the prefrontal cortex, which are pivotal for memory formation and cognitive functions. Estrogen interacts with these receptors and facilitates various brain activities, including the growth and maintenance of synaptic connections, which are vital for learning and memory.

Furthermore, fluctuating estrogen levels, especially around menopause, significantly impact cognitive abilities. The decline in estrogen levels during menopause can lead to memory impairments and increase the risk of age-related cognitive decline and dementia in women. This decline affects the brain's ability to maintain effective neuronal connections, contributing to memory lapses and cognitive challenges many women experience during this phase.

### What is the role of hormones in memory decline? How is this different between men and women?

Hormones play a pivotal role in memory function, and their influence on memory decline varies significantly between men and women. This difference is primarily due to the distinct hormonal profiles and changes experienced by each sex over their lifespan.

The decline in estrogen levels around menopause can lead to noticeable memory impairments. This reduction in estrogen affects neuronal connectivity and plasticity, leading to changes in cognitive functions.

Research has also indicated that women who experience early menopause or have lower lifetime exposure to estrogen may have an increased risk of cognitive decline later in life. Additionally, other menopausal symptoms like hot flashes and sleep disturbances can indirectly impact memory and cognitive function.

It's fascinating to see how sex hormones can have such a significant impact on neurological function including conditions like epilepsy.

## Sarita Maturu, DO, Board Director at My Epilepsy Story

*Dr. Sarita Maturu is an epileptologist and clinical assistant professor of neurology at Ohio State Wexner Medical Center. My Epilepsy Story is a nonprofit that aims to address disparities in the diagnosis of epilepsy among women and girls, striving to provide unbiased information and resources to those affected by epilepsy. Episode 198 aired March 1, 2023.*

### What is epilepsy, and how does it affect women differently?

Epilepsy is a neurological disorder characterized by recurrent, unprovoked seizures, which are sudden bursts of electrical activity in the brain that disrupt normal brain function. Epilepsy affects one in twenty-six people and can occur at any age. While epilepsy affects both men and women, there are unique considerations for women due to hormonal influences and reproductive health.

Hormonal fluctuations, particularly those related to the menstrual cycle, can impact seizure frequency and severity in women. This is known as catamenial epilepsy, where some women experience an increase in seizure activity around their menstrual periods due to changes in estrogen and progesterone levels. Estrogen tends to have a proconvulsive effect, increasing the likelihood of seizures, while progesterone has a more protective, anticonvulsant effect.

Moreover, women with epilepsy face specific challenges related to contraception, pregnancy, and menopause. Certain antiepileptic drugs can interact with hormonal contraceptives, reducing their effectiveness and raising concerns about unplanned pregnancies. During pregnancy, managing epilepsy becomes more complex as we balance the need to control seizures against potential risks to the fetus from medication exposure.

In terms of treatment, women with epilepsy must work closely with their healthcare providers to choose the right medication that minimizes risks while effectively managing their seizures. This often involves a personalized approach considering individual health needs, potential drug interactions, and lifestyle factors.

As women approach menopause, changes in hormonal levels can again affect their epilepsy. Some may experience a decrease in seizure frequency due to the drop in estrogen levels, while others might see fluctuations in seizure patterns during the perimenopausal phase.

## Tell us more about why female epilepsy patients need to coordinate with their ob-gyn for medication.

Epilepsy patients, particularly women, must coordinate their seizure medication with their ob-gyn and consider their overall female health for several key reasons. First, the interaction between anti-seizure medications and hormonal birth control can significantly impact contraceptive efficacy. Some anti-seizure medications can accelerate the metabolism of hormonal contraceptives, rendering them less effective or ineffective, thereby increasing the risk of unintended pregnancy. This necessitates careful selection of both seizure medication and contraceptive methods to ensure both are effective and do not interfere with each other.

Second, pregnancy management is crucial for women with epilepsy. Certain anti-seizure medications can have teratogenic effects, posing risks to the developing fetus. It's essential for women with epilepsy who are pregnant or planning to become pregnant to be on medications that are safest for pregnancy. This might involve adjusting medications before conception to minimize risks to both the mother and the baby.

Third, somc anti-seizure medications can affect bone health by accelerating bone turnover or contributing to osteopenia and osteoporosis. Since women are generally at higher risk for these conditions, selecting appropriate epilepsy treatment that minimizes the impact on bone density is particularly important for female patients.

Given these considerations, women with epilepsy must work closely with their healthcare providers, including neurologists and ob-gyns, to ensure their treatment plan is optimized for their neurological and reproductive health needs. This collaborative approach helps in managing epilepsy effectively while also addressing the unique health considerations of women, ensuring better outcomes and quality of life.

## Bone

### Cheryl Birch Hostinak, Executive Director at American Bone Health

*American Bone Health teaches people how to build and keep strong and healthy bones for life with practical and up-to-date information and resources to engage, educate, and empower them to prevent bone loss, osteoporosis, and fractures. Episode 160 aired March 21, 2022.*

#### What is bone health?

Bones play a crucial role in our overall health, not just as the structure that supports our bodies, but also as living tissues involved in vital processes like blood cell production. Bone health is different for men and women primarily due to hormonal differences—particularly estrogen in women—which significantly impacts bone density.

In women, bone health is closely linked to the menstrual cycle and changes dramatically with menopause. The loss of estrogen during menopause accelerates bone loss, increasing the risk of osteoporosis. This is why women are generally more susceptible to osteoporosis than men.

Osteoporosis is characterized by weakened bones, increasing the risk of fractures, and it's one of the most common bone conditions in women.

Another key aspect is that women reach their peak bone mass around thirty, after which it gradually declines. This makes it crucial for women to focus on building strong bones during their youth through a balanced diet rich in calcium and vitamin D, and regular weight-bearing exercise.

## What are the current standards of care for bone health?

The current standards of care for bone health involve a multifaceted approach that includes preventive and therapeutic strategies. First, preventive care is crucial and centers around lifestyle choices. This includes adequate calcium and vitamin D intake, regular weight-bearing and muscle-strengthening exercises, and maintaining a healthy lifestyle by avoiding smoking and limiting alcohol consumption. These measures are essential for building and maintaining bone density, especially in women.

Screening is also a key component of standard care. Women are typically recommended to undergo bone density tests (DEXA scans) starting around the age of sixty-five, or earlier if they have risk factors like a family history of osteoporosis, early menopause, or a history of bone fractures. However, there's a growing recognition of the need for earlier screening and intervention, particularly in women who experience early menopause or have other risk factors.

For those diagnosed with osteoporosis or at high risk, the standard care includes pharmacological treatments. Medications like bisphosphonates are commonly prescribed to slow bone loss; in some cases, medications that help build bone mass are used.

One of the major challenges in bone health for women is the underdiagnosis and undertreatment of osteoporosis. Many women are unaware of their bone health status until they suffer a fracture. Additionally, the onset of menopause significantly accelerates bone loss due to the decrease in estrogen, making postmenopausal women particularly vulnerable to osteoporosis and fractures.

Another challenge is adherence to preventive measures and treatment. Many women may not consistently follow through with the recommended lifestyle changes or medication regimes due to various reasons, including side effects or lack of awareness about the importance of these measures.

# Heart

## Amrita Karve, MD, Cofounder and Codirector at Women's Heart Program

*The Women's Heart Program initiative aims to increase awareness of heart disease in women, striving to improve women's health outcomes by decreasing disparities in diagnosis and treatment.*
*Episode 115 aired May 21, 2021.*

### How is heart disease different in men and women?

The differences between female and male heart disease are both subtle and significant, and understanding these differences is crucial for effective diagnosis and treatment. One of the primary distinctions lies in the way heart disease manifests in women compared to men.

First, women often experience different symptoms of heart disease and heart attacks than men. While chest pain is the most common symptom for both sexes, women are more likely to experience atypical symptoms such as fatigue, shortness of breath, nausea, and pain in the back, neck, or jaw.

These subtler symptoms can lead to misdiagnosis or delayed treatment, as they may not be immediately recognized as signs of heart disease.

Additionally, the type of heart disease can differ between sexes. Women are more likely to suffer from microvascular disease, which affects the smaller arteries in the heart. This condition can be challenging to diagnose with traditional tests that focus on larger coronary arteries, more commonly affected in men. Men, on the other hand, are more likely to develop obstructions in the major coronary arteries.

Another key difference is the impact of risk factors. Certain risk factors, such as high blood pressure and diabetes, tend to have a more significant impact on heart disease risk in women than in men. Moreover, conditions related to pregnancy, such as gestational diabetes or preeclampsia, can increase a woman's risk of developing heart disease later in life. Menopause also plays a role in increasing heart disease risk in women due to the decline in protective estrogen levels.

Last, there's the issue of representation in research. Historically, heart disease studies have predominantly focused on men, leading to a gap in understanding how the condition affects women. This lack of data can affect everything from prevention strategies to treatment protocols.

**Is cardiology adequately treating female heart disease?**

Cardiology has made significant strides, but there's still a long way to go in adequately treating female hearts. One of the main challenges is that heart disease in women often presents differently than in men, leading to underdiagnosis and undertreatment. Women might experience subtler symptoms, or symptoms that don't align with the classic signs of a heart attack, which are more commonly associated with men.

Additionally, there's a lack of representation of women in clinical trials for heart disease. This gap in research means that treatments and medications are often not as tailored to women as they should be. The physiology of women's hearts and how diseases manifest in them can be different, which needs more recognition and understanding in the medical community.

Another challenge is the need for more female cardiologists. As a male-dominated field, cardiology often needs more female perspective in practice and research. Women patients sometimes feel more comfortable and heard when discussing their health with female physicians, which can be crucial in heart disease where early diagnosis and treatment can make a significant difference.

Furthermore, societal factors play a role, too. Women often prioritize family and others' health over their own, leading to late or missed diagnoses of heart conditions. So, cardiology needs not just medical but also social change—more awareness among women about the importance of heart health and more encouragement for them to seek timely medical care.

## Gut

### Robynne Chutkan, MD, FASGE, Founder at Digestive Center for Wellness

*Dr. Robynne Chutkan is a well-recognized board-certified gastroenterologist and the author of numerous books on digestive health, including The Anti-Viral Gut, Gutbliss, The Microbiome Solution, and The Bloat Cure. She is dedicated to tackling digestive issues through managing the microbiome. Episode 143 aired November 23, 2021.*

## How are female and male gastrointestinal tracts different?

Women's and men's gastrointestinal tracts are anatomically different in several significant ways, impacting health and the manifestation of certain conditions. First, women's colons are about ten centimeters longer than men's, which is thought to aid in fluid absorption for childbearing. This extra length results in a more convoluted pathway, likened to a slinky, making gastrointestinal navigation during procedures like colonoscopies more challenging in women compared to the simpler, more direct layout often found in men.

Additionally, women's pelvic structures differ from men's, being deeper and wider to accommodate childbirth. This anatomical difference not only influences the positioning and movement of the gastrointestinal tract but also affects bowel movement patterns, potentially contributing to the higher prevalence of bloating and constipation observed in women.

Hormonal variations play a critical role as well, with testosterone contributing to a stronger, tighter abdominal wall in men. In contrast, women, having less testosterone, may have a more pliable abdominal wall, allowing the colon to bulge more and potentially exacerbating feelings of bloating.

## How do female hormones change how the gastrointestinal tract functions?

Female hormones significantly influence the gastrointestinal tract's function, creating a distinctive pattern in bowel movements, particularly in relation to menstrual cycles and menopause. Estrogen and progesterone, the primary female hormones, fluctuate throughout the menstrual cycle, impacting gut motility, the secretion of digestive enzymes, and the microbiome composition. These hormonal variations can lead to changes in bowel movement consistency and frequency, often observed as period-related constipation or diarrhea. It's common for women to experience looser stools or increased bowel activity around their periods due to the surge in prostaglandins, which stimulate muscle contractions in the uterus and can affect the bowels similarly.

As for menopause, it brings about a permanent shift in hormone levels, notably a decrease in estrogen, which can alter gut function. Many women report increased instances of bloating and constipation during menopause, attributed to hormonal changes that slow down the gastrointestinal tract. Additionally, the general decrease in bodily moisture associated with menopause can also affect the intestines, leading to drier stools and constipation. Understanding these hormonal influences on the gastrointestinal system is crucial for managing symptoms effectively and maintaining gut health during these transitional periods in a woman's life.

## Blood

### Ariela Marshall, MD Hematologist at University of Minnesota

*Dr. Ariela Marshall specializes in thrombosis and hemostasis (bleeding and clotting) disorders in women. Episode 212 aired June 7, 2023.*

#### How do blood disorders differ between men and women?

Bleeding and clotting disorders manifest differently between men and women due to various biological and hormonal factors. In women, hormonal fluctuations across their life stages, from menstruation to menopause, significantly influence both bleeding and clotting tendencies. For instance, conditions like Von Willebrand Disease, a common bleeding disorder, can be more prominent in women due to menstrual bleeding. Heavy menstrual bleeding is often the first sign of such disorders, which can go unnoticed or underdiagnosed.

On the other hand, men might experience these disorders differently, often diagnosed in situations like trauma or surgery where bleeding challenges become apparent. Furthermore, women face unique risks during pregnancy and while using hormonal contraceptives, which can increase the likelihood of clotting disorders like deep vein thrombosis.

Treatment approaches also differ. For bleeding disorders, women often need management strategies that address menstrual and reproductive health aspects, alongside standard hemostatic therapies. In clotting disorders, careful consideration is given to the choice of anticoagulants, especially during pregnancy and in women on hormonal contraceptives, to balance the risks of clotting with potential side effects.

#### Are hematologists adequately trained in women's health?

The training of hematologists in women's health varies considerably and can often be insufficient in addressing the unique needs of female patients. This gap in training can lead to significant consequences in the management of blood disorders in women. For example, conditions like heavy menstrual bleeding, which can be a symptom of an underlying hematologic issue, might be overlooked or not adequately addressed in hematologic practice. This oversight can delay diagnosis and treatment, affecting a woman's quality of life and health outcomes.

Moreover, women face unique hematologic challenges, particularly during different life stages such as pregnancy and menopause. The lack of focused training in these areas can result in suboptimal management of blood disorders during these critical times. For instance, the risk of clotting disorders increases during pregnancy, and without adequate knowledge, hematologists might miss early signs or fail to provide appropriate prophylactic measures.

The consequences of inadequate training in women's health are also evident in research and clinical trials, where historically, the specific needs and responses of female patients have been underrepresented. This gap has led to a lack of comprehensive data on how certain blood disorders and their treatments affect women differently than men.

In terms of outcomes, there can be differences between male and female hematology patients, not just due to biological factors but also because of these disparities in training and awareness. Women might experience delayed diagnoses or receive treatments that are less tailored to their physiological needs, leading to different, and sometimes less favorable, outcomes compared to male patients.

Therefore, it is imperative to integrate women's health more thoroughly into hematologic training and practice. By doing so, we can ensure that female patients receive more personalized, effective care and improve overall outcomes in hematologic disorders.

* * *

The chapter on nonuterine health illuminates the crucial need for a broader perspective on women's health that extends beyond reproductive concerns, casting a spotlight on critical areas like brain, bone, and cardiovascular health where gender disparities have profound implications. We've explored the compelling evidence that conditions like osteoporosis and Alzheimer's disease disproportionately impact women. Yet, research and treatment protocols have not always reflected this reality, often leading to underdiagnosis or inadequate care. This systemic oversight underscores the urgency of integrating a gender lens into medical research and healthcare practices. As we advocate for more inclusive research and equitable healthcare practices, the ultimate goal is to ensure that all aspects of women's health are addressed with the depth, nuance, and urgency they require. This shift toward a more comprehensive understanding of women's health will improve outcomes for women and enrich our overall approach to healthcare by ensuring that it is informed, inclusive, and just.

# Chapter 15
# Unique Challenges

**IN THE BURGEONING REALM OF WOMEN'S HEALTH,** innovators and entrepreneurs are not just introducing new products and services, but they are charting previously unexplored territories, laying down the foundational infrastructure for an entirely new industry. This pioneering journey is fraught with significant challenges, chief among them the daunting task of dismantling and rebuilding the patriarchal frameworks that have long dictated the status quo. As we venture forward, the mission extends beyond mere innovation—it's a transformative crusade aimed at redefining existing paradigms and challenging deeply ingrained assumptions. Incorporating sex and gender as critical variables requires a seismic shift in perspective, a process that, while necessary, promises to be both complex and time-consuming. The path ahead is uncharted and demanding, yet it holds the promise of reshaping the future of healthcare to cater to the needs of all women inclusively.

In its nascent stages, the FemTech industry undeniably catered to the health needs of the most affluent and privileged segments of society, mirroring the early patterns of feminist movements that predominantly centered around the experiences and needs of White women. This focus reflected and perpetuated the disparities and exclusions inherent in broader societal structures. Products and solutions initially designed by and for this demographic overlooked the diverse health concerns and cultural contexts of women from various races and ethnic backgrounds. However, today, we witness a vibrant expansion of the industry, embracing a wide array of products and solutions catering to women's health needs across different races, ethnicities, socioeconomic status, sexuality, and more.

In the grand tapestry of design and infrastructure, it's increasingly clear that women's needs and experiences have been an afterthought if considered at all. Research indicating that women take on average twice as long as men in restrooms due to insufficient facilities is just the tip of the iceberg.[177] This systemic oversight extends into professional realms, including the legislative efficiency of female lawmakers hindered by inadequate restroom access near the United States House floor, remedied only recently.

The realm of surgical tools and operating rooms further exemplifies this disparity. As more women enter fields traditionally dominated by men, such as surgery, the ergonomic challenges they face due to equipment designed for the average male physique become increasingly evident. The design of surgical instruments, operating room layouts, and even the protective gear intended to shield surgeons from radiation fail to account for the physical diversity of the workforce, especially women. Female surgeons are more likely to experience discomfort, pain, or injury from using tools and equipment ill-suited to their body sizes and shapes.[178] This not only affects their personal health and career longevity but also raises concerns about patient care quality. Surgical gloves not fitting, operating beds not adjusting to optimal heights, and protective gear not adequately shielding female anatomy from radiation are stark indicators of a profession—and indeed, a society—that has yet to fully embrace inclusivity in its design philosophy.

The implications of these design oversights are profound, affecting women's ability to work and live comfortably and highlighting the economic and health costs of such neglect. When female professionals must make do with tools and environments not tailored to their needs, it's clear that the systems and products around them are yet to fully acknowledge women's rightful place in all spheres of life. This scenario underscores the necessity for FemTech and other industries to innovate solutions and critically reevaluate and adjust existing infrastructures to accommodate the diversity of women's bodies and needs. As we strive toward a more inclusive society, acknowledging and addressing these disparities head-on is not just a matter of fairness but a crucial step toward unlocking the full potential of half the population.

The sexualization of female bodies and the societal taboo surrounding natural biological processes has led to significant censorship of female health, underpinned by a perception of inappropriateness. This phenomenon is starkly evident in the realms of social media and advertising, where women's health content often faces unjust classification and removal. For instance, a Center for Intimacy Justice report highlighted that Meta's policies categorize discussions on women's health as akin to adult products or services, thereby breaching community standards. This discriminatory practice starkly contrasts with the leniency shown toward male sexual wellness advertisements, which frequently navigate these platforms with ease and without the threat of censorship. Such disparities not only reflect the ingrained sexualization of women's bodies but also the systemic sidelining of female-centric health issues, creating barriers to important health education and fostering a culture of silence and shame around women's natural biological processes.

Moreover, the stigma and censorship surrounding women's health have tangible consequences on the accessibility of information and support for women. Platforms that once promised to democratize access to health knowledge now often serve as gatekeepers, filtering and policing content related to women's health under the guise of propriety. This censorship extends to critical postpartum care and menstrual health, with impactful stories and advertisements—like the rejected Frida Mom commercial intended for the Oscars—being deemed too graphic or explicit for public consumption. By contrast, content that aligns with traditional male narratives and sexual health is seldom subjected to the same scrutiny, highlighting a glaring bias in how we, as a society, regulate and value health information based on gender.

The consequences of this systemic censorship are profound, limiting women's ability to share and access vital information about their own bodies and health. The fight for space and voice in the public domain by companies like Dame Products, which faced discrimination by the New York Metropolitan Transportation Authority (MTA) over advertisements for women's pleasure products, underscores the broader struggle against the sexualization and censorship of female health. Such challenges not only stifle innovation and awareness in female health technology and services but also perpetuate a culture of shame and ignorance. Breaking these barriers is essential for fostering a society that values and supports women's health equitably, recognizing it not as a niche or inappropriate topic but as a fundamental aspect of human health deserving of open discussion, research, and investment.

As we reflect on the journey of women's health innovation, it's evident that the path is fraught with systemic obstacles rooted in a long-standing tradition of gender bias and societal norms. Yet, amid these challenges, there is a resilient push toward breaking down the barriers and redefining the narrative around women's health. The journey ahead requires a collective effort to dismantle these patriarchal constructs and embrace a more inclusive and equitable approach to health innovation. By acknowledging and addressing these challenges, we can pave the way for a future where women's health is not sidelined but celebrated and supported, fostering a society that genuinely respects and uplifts all aspects of female well-being.

## Government and Policy

### Kimberly Haven, Founder and Director at Reproductive Justice Inside

*Kimberly Haven is a prominent figure in many women's movements, especially advocating for the rights of incarcerated and formerly incarcerated women, drawing from her own experiences of incarceration. Episode 202 aired March 29, 2023.*

**What is women's healthcare like for incarcerated women in the US?**

Women's healthcare in US prisons is grossly inadequate and often fails to address the unique needs of incarcerated women.

Menstruation is another area where the needs of incarcerated women are frequently overlooked. Access to menstrual products is limited, and women often have to resort to makeshift solutions, which can lead to health risks. Some prisons provide basic sanitary products, often insufficient in quantity and quality.

Access to reproductive healthcare, including prenatal care, is often limited and inconsistent across different states. Childbirth in prison is a challenging experience. Some states have protocols for pregnant women, but these vary widely. In many cases, the support and medical care provided are minimal, and women often go through childbirth without the presence of a loved one or adequate emotional support. Post-delivery, babies are usually separated from their mothers, which can have lasting psychological effects. And the prison healthcare system is not set up to address challenges like postpartum depression.

Breastfeeding and expressing breast milk in prison are complex issues. While some facilities might allow it, the support for breastfeeding, like providing breast pumps or facilitating the storage and transportation of breast milk (like through initiatives such as Boober, a nonprofit that helps women get their breast milk to their babies while they are incarcerated), is not standard across all prisons. This lack of support can impede a mother's ability to maintain a bond with her child and provide the best nutrition.

Menopause in prison is another area that's largely ignored. Incarcerated women going through menopause often do not receive adequate healthcare or support to manage symptoms like hot flashes. Access to hormonal treatments or even basic amenities like fans to alleviate discomfort can be limited.

### Why is healthcare for women in prisons so inadequate?

The inadequacy of healthcare for women in prisons is rooted in several systemic issues. First and foremost, the prison system was primarily designed for men and did not adequately address the unique healthcare needs of women. This oversight results in a lack of policies and practices tailored to women's health concerns, including reproductive health, mental health, and chronic diseases that disproportionately affect women.

Additionally, there's a significant lack of awareness and training among prison staff regarding women's health issues. This gap in knowledge leads to neglect and inadequate care. For example, the handling of menstruation, pregnancy, childbirth, and menopause in prisons often lacks sensitivity and medical appropriateness because the staff may not be adequately trained to address these issues.

Another factor is the systemic underfunding and overcrowding of prisons, which strains the available resources and healthcare infrastructure. This situation leads to prioritization of acute and emergency care while neglecting preventive and routine care, which is vital for women's health.

There's also a prevalent culture of indifference and sometimes hostility toward prisoners, which further exacerbates the issue. Women in prison, particularly those who are pregnant or have specific health needs, face stigma and discrimination, which can deter them from seeking necessary care.

Last, there's a lack of political will and public advocacy focused on the health rights of incarcerated women. This lack of attention results in slow or no reform in prison healthcare policies and practices.

## Heidi Morin, MSN, MBA, RN, FABCH, Founder and CEO at Parity Healthcare Analytics

*Parity Healthcare Analytics is a staffing software providing real-time data on current patients' needs, ensuring adequate nurse staffing. They aim to tackle maternal mortality rates by facilitating enough nursing staff each shift to care for unique patient needs. Episode 200 aired March 15, 2023.*

### What is so unique about staffing a maternity ward? What are the consequences of staffing inadequately?

Staffing a maternity ward is unique due to maternity care's diverse and often unpredictable nature. It involves caring for both the mother and the newborn, which requires a multifaceted approach and a wide range of skills from the nursing staff. We deal with varying stages of labor, delivery, postpartum care, and potential complications, making it one of the most challenging yet rewarding areas in nursing.

Inadequate staffing in maternity wards can have dire consequences. It's not just about numbers; it's about having skilled personnel who can respond effectively to mothers' and babies' dynamic and sometimes rapidly changing needs. When a ward is understaffed, there are several areas of concern.

The risk of missing critical signs or delayed response to emergencies increases. This can lead to adverse outcomes, including higher rates of complications, morbidity, or even mortality for mothers and babies.

Overworked staff are more prone to burnout, leading to high turnover rates. This affects the team's morale and impacts continuity of care and the overall quality of healthcare delivery.

The patient experience can significantly deteriorate in understaffed wards. Personalized care is crucial during childbirth, and when nurses are stretched thin, they cannot provide the level of care and attention each patient deserves.

**Is operating a maternity ward expensive for a hospital? What is a maternity desert?**

Operating a maternity ward is expensive, primarily due to the high level of specialized care required. Maternity wards are unique healthcare environments where the safety and well-being of two patients—the mother and the baby—are simultaneously managed. This requires not only a higher number of nursing staff compared to other wards but also staff with specialized skills in obstetrics, neonatal care, and emergency response. Additionally, the equipment and facilities needed in maternity wards, such as delivery rooms, operating rooms for cesarean sections, and neonatal intensive care units, contribute to higher operational costs.

What's concerning is the trend of maternity wards shutting down, especially in rural and underserved areas. This is often due to financial constraints. Maternity wards are not as profitable as other departments in a hospital, and when healthcare systems face budget cuts or financial decisions, maternity services are sometimes seen as expendable. This is particularly true in areas with lower population density or a higher proportion of patients relying on Medicaid, which typically reimburses at a lower rate than private insurance.

The closure of maternity wards leads to what we call *maternity deserts*. A maternity desert is an area, often rural or underserved, where there is limited or no access to maternity care services. This includes the absence of a maternity ward and a lack of obstetricians, midwives, and related healthcare providers. These deserts pose a significant risk to maternal and infant health, as they force women to travel long distances for prenatal care and delivery, which can lead to delayed or inadequate care, higher rates of complications, and adverse outcomes. The existence of maternity deserts is a growing concern in the US, reflecting broader issues of healthcare accessibility and inequality.

## Beth A. Brooke, Cochair at VERITY NOW

*VERITY (Vehicle Equity Rules in Transportation) NOW unites people to fight for equality in vehicle safety by educating on and advocating for crash testing standards that protect men and women equally, making cars safer for all. Episode 171 aired July 11, 2022.*

## What safety tools and equipment have not been optimized for women's bodies?

Automobile safety, personal protective equipment (PPE), and sports equipment have long been designed with a male-centric perspective, neglecting the anatomical and physiological differences of women. This oversight significantly affects women's safety and performance across various fields.

In the realm of automobile safety, women are 73 percent more likely to be severely injured and 17 percent more likely to die in car crashes than men. This disparity arises because Federal Motor Vehicle Safety Standards (FMVSS) are based on male crash test dummies. Despite the existence of a female crash test dummy, known as SET 50F, equipped with appropriate sensors for areas where women are more likely to sustain injuries, such as the legs and neck, it's not widely used. The United States, unlike Europe and Asia, has not yet required its use, resulting in vehicles that are less safe for women. The argument that changing standards would be cost-prohibitive is unfounded, as the adjustment would cost less than $1 per car.

Similarly, PPE in industries like firefighting, oil, and mining has historically been designed for men's bodies. This misalignment can lead to an increased risk of injury for women, as ill-fitting gear fails to provide adequate protection. For example, firefighters' gear not tailored to women's bodies can compromise their safety in dangerous environments.

Sports equipment and training regimens also often overlook the unique needs of female athletes, potentially affecting performance and increasing injury risks. An example is the lack of consideration for the menstrual cycle's impact on women's physical capabilities and injury rates, pointing to a critical need for research and innovation in training methods and equipment design for women.

The root cause of these disparities lies in a long-standing bias within design and research, where women's specific needs are overlooked or deemed too complicated to address. A lack of female representation among engineers, designers, and decision-makers in these fields perpetuates this bias. To rectify these issues, it's imperative to include more women in the design process, advocate for inclusive research and testing that considers sex as a biological variable, and demand changes to standards and practices that currently favor male anatomy. We can only ensure that women's safety and performance needs are equally prioritized through concerted effort and advocacy.

### What is VERITY NOW's mission?

VERITY NOW advocates changes to FMVSS to require female crash test dummies, like the Thor-5F, in all safety tests. This is crucial to ensuring cars are designed with the safety of both women and men in mind. Our approach involves raising public awareness about the disparity in vehicle safety and mobilizing public support to demand change. We are engaging with policymakers, leveraging data and research to illustrate the stark differences in injury and fatality rates between women and men in car crashes, and emphasizing the feasibility and cost-effectiveness of integrating female crash test dummies into standard testing protocols.

Legislative and regulatory changes are necessary for car companies to be mandated to test and optimize car safety for all bodies. This entails updating the FMVSS to include requirements for using female crash test dummies in safety tests. Public pressure and advocacy are key to achieving this, as is the support from lawmakers willing to champion these changes. It's about ensuring that vehicle design and safety testing are inclusive, reflecting the diversity of drivers and passengers. Ultimately, it's not just about compliance but valuing human life equally and recognizing that safety should not be gender biased.

## Liz Powell, MPH, Founder and President at Government to Growth (G2G) Consulting

*G2G develops and executes government-to-growth (G2G) strategies by providing comprehensive government affairs, public relations, and economic development services for businesses and nonprofits. Its primary focus is connecting innovators to the US government.*
*Episode 194 aired February 1, 2023.*

### How does policy affect women's health?

Policy profoundly impacts women's health across various dimensions, from research funding to clinical practices and access to care. A mere 11 percent of the National Institutes of Health (NIH) research funding is currently dedicated to women's health, underscoring a significant gap in our understanding and treatment of conditions disproportionately affecting women. This underfunding has systemic repercussions, limiting advancements in diagnostics, treatment, and overall care for women.

Collaboration with entities like the Office of Research on Women's Health is crucial for increasing this funding. Yet, despite such efforts, challenges persist due to structural complexities within our health systems and the distribution of research dollars. For instance, the Office of Research on Women's Health, pivotal in coordinating studies across other institutes, is hindered by its limited capacity to conduct its own research, thereby constraining its influence on broadening the scope of women's health research.

Moreover, policy can either catalyze or inhibit the development of innovative healthcare solutions. Examples include developing policy proposals to close women's health research gaps, medical training, diagnostics, and clinical care. Such initiatives necessitate a deep understanding of systemic problems and the articulation of viable solutions that can be implemented at the policy level.

Engagement with policymakers through letter-writing campaigns and direct advocacy is another avenue through which policy can be shaped to better serve women's health. These activities raise legislators' awareness about critical health issues and offer a platform for proposing evidence-based interventions. For instance, a successful campaign led to increased funding for the Office of Research on Women's Health, showcasing the potential impact of concerted advocacy efforts.

On the regulatory front, policy decisions made by bodies like the Centers for Medicare and Medicaid Services (CMS) directly influence the accessibility and affordability of healthcare services for women. The establishment of reimbursement codes, for example, determines whether and how new medical technologies and treatments can be integrated into standard care, ultimately affecting patient outcomes.

Policy intersects with every facet of women's health, from the allocation of research funds to the regulatory frameworks governing healthcare practices. The challenges are manifold, but significant strides can be made in advancing women's health outcomes through strategic advocacy, education, and direct engagement with policymakers. The journey toward equitable healthcare is complex, but with persistent effort and targeted policy interventions, we can pave the way for a more inclusive and effective healthcare system.

**How has the overturning of the right to abortion in the US affected voter turnout?**

The overturning of *Roe v. Wade* has significantly galvanized voter turnout and heightened public engagement with policy issues surrounding women's health. By stripping away the constitutional right to abortion, this landmark decision has not only mobilized individuals across the nation to register to vote but also motivated them to participate in the political process actively. In the aftermath, we observed a remarkable surge in women registering to vote in many states, indicating a collective determination to influence policy decisions that directly impact women's autonomy over their bodies.

This increased political activation reflects a broader awakening to the critical importance of safeguarding women's health rights through legislative means. While the assumption that all women vote uniformly on this issue does not hold true—given the diversity of opinions and beliefs—it's evident that the decision has catalyzed broader engagement with health policy matters.

Moreover, the decision's timing, just ahead of key elections, magnified its impact on voter mobilization. Clearly, the loss of this right, which many had taken for granted for almost half a century, has awakened a significant portion of the electorate to the urgent need for action. It has underscored the importance of voting and engaging continuously with elected representatives, advocating for policies that protect and advance women's health rights.

The reaction to the *Dobbs* decision underscores a profound shift, illuminating the critical role of policy in shaping health outcomes and rights. It serves as a stark reminder that the fight for women's health rights is far from over and that active, informed participation in the democratic process is essential for effecting meaningful change.

## Jackie Rotman, Founder and CEO at Center for Intimacy Justice

*The Center for Intimacy Justice believes in catalyzing greater technological innovation and investment, education, and cultural understanding of female sexual health and in building a culture of greater equity, agency, and well-being. Episode 167 aired June 6, 2022.*

### How and why are women's health digital media being censored?

The censorship of women's health advertisements is a profound issue that significantly impacts the FemTech industry. These ads are being systematically banned or restricted on major ad platforms like Facebook, Instagram, and Google due to policies that inappropriately classify women's health and sexual wellness products as adult content. This censorship creates substantial barriers for FemTech companies striving to reach their audience and disseminate valuable health information.

For instance, our research at the Center for Intimacy Justice, which surveyed sixty women's health companies, revealed that 100 percent of these companies had experienced ad rejections from Meta platforms, with 50 percent having their entire accounts suspended at some point. This is not a small issue but a pervasive barrier affecting the entire FemTech sector.

The reasons behind these bans are multifaceted but largely stem from outdated and discriminatory policies that view women's health through a sexualized lens, irrespective of the educational or health-focused nature of the content. Products and services related to menopause, menstrual health, sexual wellness, and even breastfeeding are frequently flagged and categorized alongside sexually explicit material. This misclassification is largely driven by automated algorithms that lack the nuance to distinguish between health-related content and adult content.

Additionally, there's a glaring double standard in treatment of men's and women's health products. For example, ads promoting erectile dysfunction medications have been allowed and even mainstreamed, while ads for women's health products addressing equally valid medical concerns are censored. This not only stifles FemTech companies' ability to grow and reach their potential customers but also contributes to the broader societal issue of silencing conversations around women's health.

The impact of this censorship is substantial. It impedes the growth of FemTech companies by limiting their marketing reach and potential for customer engagement. It also affects their financial trajectories, making it challenging to attract venture capital funding. Beyond the direct impact on companies, this censorship deprives individuals of access to critical health information and products that could significantly improve their quality of life.

## What is the Center for Intimacy Justice?

The Center for Intimacy Justice is the first organization to address censorship and discrimination against sexual wellness and women's health companies in business and advertising. We work on the front lines to advocate for the rights of FemTech and sexual wellness companies, ensuring they can advertise their products and services freely, just like businesses in any other sector.

Our work involves a multi-pronged approach to changing censorship rules. First, we conduct research and publish reports highlighting censorship's extent and impact on women's health and sexual wellness companies. Our findings have caught the attention of major media outlets and even Congress, raising awareness and sparking conversations about the need for change.

Second, we engage directly with policymakers and platforms to advocate for clearer, more equitable advertising policies. Platforms like Facebook, Instagram, and Google can swiftly change these rules if they prioritize them. Our engagement aims to demonstrate the importance of this issue and the positive impact that reforming these policies can have on society at large.

Changing these censorship rules requires a concerted effort from multiple stakeholders. It's not just about policy reform within ad platforms but also about societal change in how we view and discuss women's health. Platforms must update their algorithms and policy guidelines to distinguish between adult content and legitimate health information. This involves recognizing FemTech advertisements' educational and health-focused nature and ensuring they are not unjustly categorized or banned.

Others can help in this fight by raising awareness, supporting organizations working on these issues, and demanding change from platforms and policymakers. Businesses affected by these policies can share their stories, contributing to a larger narrative that underscores the need for reform. Consumers and the general public can amplify this issue through social media, engagements with elected officials, and supporting FemTech companies facing these challenges.

Together, through collective action and advocacy, we can push for a world where conversations about women's health are not silenced but embraced and supported, enabling a healthier and more informed society.

## Diversity and Inclusion

### Rasha Babikir, MBBS, MBA, Director at Cedar Health Research

*Cedar Health Research is a clinical trial site network utilizing AI to match diverse populations with clinical trials to address research gaps in underrepresented groups. Episode 196 aired February 15, 2023.*

#### Why were women excluded from clinical trials?

The exclusion of women from clinical trials, particularly those of childbearing potential, was primarily due to the thalidomide tragedy that occurred in the late 1950s and early 1960s. Thalidomide was a drug initially used as a sedative or tranquilizer, but it was later prescribed for managing morning sickness in pregnant women. Unfortunately, the drug led to severe teratogenic effects, causing thousands of babies to be born with congenital defects, including limb malformations and, in some cases, brain damage.

As a result of this tragedy, the FDA and other regulatory bodies became highly cautious about the involvement of women of childbearing age in clinical trials. The fear was that a similar incident could occur if pregnant women or women who might become pregnant were exposed to experimental drugs without fully understanding the risks to their unborn children. Consequently, in 1977, a mandate was issued that effectively banned the inclusion of women of childbearing potential in clinical trials. This was done with the ethical aim of protecting them.

This decision aimed to prevent potential harm to fetuses due to the unknown effects of new drugs or treatments being tested in these trials. It was a protective measure, but it also led to a significant gap in medical research, as women's specific health needs and responses to various treatments were not adequately studied for many years.

This mandate was only revised in 1993. The realization that drugs could react differently in men and women and the lack of women-specific data led to a change in policy. The new guidelines still required strict protocols to ensure the safety of women, especially those who might become pregnant, but they allowed for their inclusion in clinical research. This change was crucial in understanding gender differences in medicine and ensuring women received effective and safe medical treatments.

**What is the current state of female involvement in clinical trials?**

The current state of female involvement in clinical trials has improved significantly since the 1990s. Women are now more actively included in clinical research, which is crucial for understanding gender differences in disease manifestation and treatment responses. However, there are still challenges. Women, particularly those of childbearing age, are underrepresented in some areas of clinical research. This underrepresentation can be attributed to various factors, including historical biases, logistic challenges, and concerns about potential risks to reproductive health.

One key barrier to female participation is the lack of awareness about the importance of clinical trials and how they contribute to medical advancements. Educational campaigns targeting women, explaining the safety measures in place, and highlighting the potential benefits of participating in trials can be effective.

Recruitment strategies should be tailored to address women's specific concerns and needs. This includes providing clear information about the study, its risks, benefits, and protective measures for women, especially those who are pregnant or might become pregnant.

Offering flexible scheduling options and providing support services, such as childcare and transportation, can help women balance their participation in a trial with their other responsibilities.

Building trust within female communities is crucial. This can be achieved by engaging with women's groups, healthcare providers primarily serving women, and other community leaders who can advocate for clinical trial participation.

It's important to address diversity in clinical trials, not just regarding gender, but also considering racial, ethnic, and socioeconomic diversity. Diverse participation ensures that clinical research findings apply to a wider population.

## Marissa Fayer, MBA, Founder and CEO at HERhealthEQ

*The HERhealthEQ team is driven by a desire to see fewer women face the choice between their own healthcare and putting food on the tables of their families. Our mission is to improve women's health in developing countries by providing access to medical devices and equipment, creating an equitable standard of care. Episode 117 aired May 24, 2021.*

## What challenges do developing countries face when it comes to medical equipment?

In developing countries, women's healthcare faces numerous challenges, including limited access to essential medical equipment. This lack of resources significantly impacts the diagnosis, treatment, and management of noncommunicable diseases among women. For instance, the infrastructure in many of these areas may not support the power requirements of advanced medical devices, making it challenging to utilize equipment like mammography machines without additional converters or upgrades.

To address these challenges, our organization conducts thorough site surveys to understand each location's specific needs and limitations. Despite these efforts, some places cannot support certain types of equipment due to infrastructural constraints. This reality underscores the urgent need for equipment designed with the developing world's context in mind.

The scarcity of medical equipment severely affects women's health in these regions. For example, we have focused on providing ultrasound machines, fetal monitors, and devices for detecting and treating cervical cancer, such as colposcopes and thermal ablation equipment. These tools are crucial for women's health yet are often inaccessible in low-resource settings.

The impact of our work is measurable. To date, we have deployed $71,000 worth of medical equipment, impacting over 41,000 women across six countries. However, our goal is ambitious—we aim to impact the lives of one million women by the end of 2025. This requires deploying over 200 pieces of equipment, emphasizing the scale of the need for medical resources in these communities.

The lack of medical equipment affects individual health outcomes and has broader implications for education and economic empowerment. Women are often the primary caregivers in their families, and their ill health can lead to increased school dropout rates among girls. Furthermore, healthy women contribute significantly to their families and communities, with 90 percent of a woman's income reinvested into her family, compared to 35 percent of a man's.

## Tell us about HERhealthEQ.

HERhealthEQ is a nonprofit organization committed to enhancing healthcare for women in developing countries by equipping them with essential medical devices. Our mission is rooted in the belief that improving women's health is foundational to community development and gender equity in healthcare. Through our efforts, we focus on addressing noncommunicable diseases, a significant health burden for women in these regions, by providing needed medical equipment and support.

To date, HERhealthEQ has made notable strides by deploying medical equipment across several countries, including under-resourced areas in the Caribbean, Africa, and parts of Asia. Our projects have supplied a range of essential medical devices, from ultrasound machines and fetal monitors to innovative solutions for detecting and treating cervical cancer. This initiative has facilitated vital health services and empowered women to pursue healthier, more productive lives, significantly impacting their communities' economic and social fabric. Our vision for the future is bold and clear: to impact the lives of one million women by the end of 2025.

## Harpreet Nagra, PhD, Former Vice President of Behavior Science at One Drop

*One Drop is a precision health company that combines continuous diagnostics, predictive analytics, and machine learning in an award-winning, digital solution to deliver cost-saving outcomes for people with diabetes and other chronic conditions. Episode 156 aired February 20, 2022.*

### What is cultural sensitivity? What role does it play in digital health?

Cultural sensitivity, or perhaps more aptly, cultural humility, refers to recognizing, respecting, and addressing individuals' diverse cultural backgrounds and experiences. This approach emphasizes openness to learning from mistakes, acknowledging when we don't know something, and committing to continuous improvement in understanding and integrating the cultural contexts of all stakeholders. In the digital health sphere, cultural humility is vital to creating genuinely inclusive solutions that meet the varied needs of a diverse population.

The digital health industry is currently on a journey toward greater cultural sensitivity, but considerable work must be done. The baseline databases and algorithms driving many digital health solutions often reflect inherent biases, primarily because they are built on data that lacks diversity in race, gender, ethnicity, and socioeconomic status. This lack of diversity in data leads to solutions that may not be fully applicable or beneficial to all populations, potentially exacerbating existing health disparities.

The consequences of not being culturally sensitive in digital health are significant. First, it can lead to the development of products and services that are not effective for diverse populations, thereby failing to address or even worsening health disparities. For example, a survey mentioned in the conversation highlighted that 68 percent of young technologists felt uncomfortable in their workplaces due to their gender, ethnicity, socioeconomic background, or a hidden condition. This discomfort can lead to a talent drain, where individuals leave their positions for environments where they feel more valued and included. This not only hampers innovation but also prevents the creation of digital health solutions that cater to the needs of a diverse user base.

Moreover, a lack of cultural sensitivity can alienate potential users who feel that their specific needs and contexts are not considered or understood. Digital health solutions that fail to account for cultural differences in health perceptions, practices, and challenges might not be adopted by those who could benefit from them the most, thereby limiting their impact.

## How can digital health apps be culturally sensitive?

Digital health apps must embrace cultural sensitivity by ensuring their design, development, and deployment processes are inclusive and respectful of diverse cultural backgrounds. This involves utilizing data representing a broad spectrum of races, genders, ethnicities, and socioeconomic backgrounds to inform algorithms and databases, thus preventing biases and ensuring the app's relevance across different populations. The design of interfaces and user experiences must be accessible to and resonate with a wide audience, incorporating language options, culturally relevant imagery and content, and accessibility features to make digital health apps universally usable.

Engaging with communities from various cultural backgrounds during the development process can provide valuable insights into the unique needs and preferences of different groups, fostering more effective and widely accepted solutions. Investing in cultural competence training for teams enhances their understanding and sensitivity toward cultural differences, helping prevent unconscious biases from influencing product development and customer service. Implementing mechanisms to collect and respond to feedback from diverse user groups allows for continuous learning from user experiences, guiding the evolution of the app to be more culturally sensitive over time.

Being culturally sensitive significantly benefits digital health businesses by expanding their market reach, tapping into wider markets, and attracting a broader user base. It leads to higher satisfaction by meeting the specific needs of users, increasing usage, and encouraging positive word of mouth. Culturally sensitive apps can better address health inequities, positioning the company as a leader in equitable healthcare solutions. Demonstrating respect and understanding of cultural diversity enhances trust in the brand, fostering long-term user engagement. To be culturally sensitive, digital health companies must commit to ongoing learning, adaptation, and engagement with diverse communities, fostering innovation and business growth while making healthcare more inclusive and equitable.

## Data Privacy

### Laura Lázaro Cabrera, LLM, Former Senior Legal Officer at Privacy International

*Privacy International is a nonprofit organization that advocates for laws protecting privacy. It promotes litigation efforts and research to prevent governments and corporations from interfering with privacy.*
*Episode Bonus 11 aired July 15, 2022.*

**Why do women's health companies and female users of digital health need to be aware of data privacy?**

The importance of data privacy in women's digital health cannot be overstated. With the growing use of technology in health and wellness, especially in FemTech, a significant amount of sensitive personal data is being collected, processed, and potentially shared. This data can include menstrual cycles, sexual activity, fertility information, pregnancy, and even more personal aspects like mood swings or contraceptive use. The need for heightened privacy awareness stems from several key concerns.

First, the sensitivity of this data cannot be underestimated. Information about a woman's reproductive health is incredibly personal and, in many contexts, can have serious implications if mishandled or exposed. For example, in regions where reproductive rights are contested or restricted, such data could potentially be used against women in legal or social contexts.

Second, there's the issue of consent and control. Many users may not fully understand how their data is being used, who it's being shared with, or how it's protected. Digital health companies must be transparent about their data practices and give users clear, understandable, and accessible ways to control their data. This includes the ability to opt in or out of data sharing and access, correct their data, or delete their data.

Last, the evolving legal landscape around data privacy, such as the General Data Protection Regulation (GDPR) in Europe and various state laws in the US, makes it crucial for companies to stay compliant to avoid legal repercussions and to maintain user trust. In an era where data breaches are increasingly common, robust data security practices are essential to protect sensitive health information.

### How well are women's health apps handling women's health data today?

Today, handling women's health data by health apps presents a mixed picture. On the positive side, there has been growing awareness among app developers and users about the importance of data privacy and security. This is partly driven by increased public attention to data breaches and privacy concerns, as well as the implementation of stricter data protection regulations like the GDPR in Europe. As a result, many women's health apps have started to adopt better data protection practices, such as improved encryption, clearer privacy policies, and more user-friendly consent mechanisms.

However, challenges remain. Despite these improvements, significant concerns remain about how some apps collect, use, and share women's health data. For instance, issues around data sharing with third parties, particularly for advertising and analytics purposes, are still prevalent. Many apps may collect more data than necessary for their functionality, leading to potential overreach into users' privacy.

Furthermore, the diversity in quality and standards among apps is notable. While some apps demonstrate a strong commitment to protecting users' data, others may lack adequate security measures or transparency in their data practices. This inconsistency can leave users vulnerable, especially in regions with less stringent data protection laws.

Another concern is the potential use of sensitive data in ways that users might not anticipate or consent to, such as selling anonymized data to third parties, which can sometimes be reidentified.

* * *

In the dynamic landscape of women's health startups, entrepreneurs face unique challenges beyond the typical hurdles of funding and market penetration. As these pioneers strive to reshape a sector deeply entrenched in traditional, often patriarchal medical practices, they confront the critical task of dismantling long-standing biases and misconceptions that have historically sidelined women's health. This journey is not just about introducing innovative products or services; it's a broader crusade for systemic change, advocating for a profound shift in how healthcare addresses the needs of women. These challenges are compounded by the necessity to educate a market that has been historically underserved and misunderstood, requiring startups to not only sell their products but also champion the legitimacy and critical importance of focusing on women's health. Thus, while the path forward is fraught with obstacles, it promises significant social impact, potentially leading to a more inclusive and equitable healthcare landscape.

# Chapter 16
# Funding Women's Health

**IN THE DYNAMIC ECOSYSTEM OF STARTUP FUNDING,** the avenues available for securing financial backing are as diverse as they are critical. Government grants, typically offered by agencies like the NIH, provide a crucial lifeline for early stage research and development, often serving as the first vote of confidence in a startup's potential. Angel investors, individuals investing their personal money and driven by a deep belief in the founder or the proposed solution, step in to nurture early product development and market entry strategies. Powered by financial commitments from affluent families, pension funds, and endowments, venture capital firms propel startups into their growth phases, betting on those that demonstrate a strong product-market fit. Meanwhile, private equity firms target established entities, injecting substantial funds to scale operations significantly. Each of these funding mechanisms plays a pivotal role in the life cycle of a startup, catering to its evolving needs from inception to maturity.

Investing in a startup is as much an emotional decision as it is financial. Investors, whether angels or venture capitalists, look for businesses that promise lucrative exits within a decade, offering substantial returns. However, the emotional connection to the startup's mission, the problems it aims to solve, and the innovative nature of its solutions significantly influence investment decisions. This blend of financial acumen and personal enthusiasm underlines the importance of investors' familiarity with the industry and their conviction in the startup's potential. It's a delicate balance, where the promise of financial returns and a deep-seated belief in the startup's value proposition play crucial roles. Unfortunately, this intricate dance of numbers and emotions often places FemTech startups at a disadvantage, primarily due to the historical male dominance in investment circles.

FemTech startups, innovating at the intersection of technology and women's health, frequently find themselves at a crossroads, struggling to ignite the same excitement among traditionally male investor groups. The challenges are manifold: a need for more representation in investment decisions, underestimation of the women's health market's size, and biases toward more familiar sectors. This misperception of FemTech as a niche and a scarcity of data on the industry's financial viability has historically deterred investors. Until recently, the successes of women's health companies were underreported, and comprehensive market research was scarce, perpetuating a cycle of misinformation and missed opportunities. The term *FemTech,* only coined in 2016 by Ida Tin, highlights the nascent recognition of the field. The resultant knowledge gap has been a significant barrier, hindering investors' ability to fully appreciate the scope and potential of innovations in women's health, thus slowing the flow of capital into an area ripe with opportunity for transformative impact.

Historically, the landscape of government funding for women's health research reveals a stark imbalance, underscoring a systemic oversight that has long permeated the scientific community. In the United States, where up to 45 percent of life sciences research garners support from federal and nonfederal government sources, the allocation toward women's health research has been disproportionately low.[179] Despite the NIH commanding a formidable $45 billion budget in fiscal year 2022, a mere $4.6 billion—a fraction of the total—was explicitly earmarked for women's health.[180,181] This discrepancy is further compounded by the absence of a dedicated institute within the NIH focused on women's health, leaving researchers to navigate other institutes to advocate for the importance of sex-specific studies. Before the landmark Sex as a Biological Variable Act of 2016, the granularity of analyzing data by sex in cellular, animal, or human studies was not a mandated aspect of research proposals, spotlighting the historical inertia against recognizing the unique dimensions of women's health in scientific inquiry.

| DISEASE | % FEMALES AFFECTED | FEMALES IMPACTED (Millions) | % of NIH 2020 BUDGET |
|---|---|---|---|
| Menopause | 85% | 140 | <0.00001% |
| Menstrual Disorders | 55% | 83 | 0.00004% |
| Fibroids | 22% | 33 | 0.001% |
| Pelvic Floor Disorder | 18% | 30 | 0.002% |
| Vulvodynia | 16% | 27 | 0.0008% |
| Endometriosis | 10% | 17 | 0.0009% |

*Figure 14: Severe underfunding of women's health research by the National Institutes of Health (NIH) as shown by the percentage of 2020 NIH budget allocated to extremely prevalent conditions and life phases of females in the United States.*[182]

This underfunding is not an anomaly confined to the United States but a global issue, with countries like Canada and the United Kingdom allocating a meager 5.9 percent of their health research grants toward studies focusing on women's health or female-specific outcomes from 2009 to 2020.[183] Such funding disparities have real-world repercussions; despite women exhibiting a 50 percent higher mortality rate following a heart attack than men, only a scant 4.5 percent of the NIH's coronary artery disease budget is dedicated to women-focused research.[184,185] The imbalance extends to the prioritization of research topics, with erectile dysfunction studies historically outnumbering those on premenstrual syndrome by a factor of five. Even in instances where research showed promising results—such as the case with sildenafil citrate's potential to alleviate menstrual pain—projects were halted due to financial constraints. This funding gap not only highlights a troubling oversight in addressing women's health issues, but it also underscores a broader societal challenge in prioritizing and investing in the health and well-being of women.

The journey of venture capital funding into women's health and FemTech has been a slow but gradually accelerating process, marked by pivotal moments and pioneering funds recognizing the vast potential within this underexplored sector. Astarte Ventures emerged as the trailblazer in 2013, becoming the first venture fund dedicated to FemTech.

However, its journey shifted focus as its general partners transitioned to operating one of their invested businesses. This initial foray set the stage for Portfolia in 2018, a novel venture initiative that sought to invest in FemTech and democratize the venture capital process for women. Through Portfolia's series of specialized funds, including their third FemTech-focused fund, they amassed the largest portfolio with forty-six investments, signaling a growing recognition of women's health as a lucrative and impactful investment opportunity. The subsequent surge in FemTech venture funds—from a mere single $10 million venture fund in 2020 to over twelve venture funds managing over $380 million by 2024, all spearheaded by women—underscores a monumental shift in the landscape, driven by a profound understanding of the need and potential for innovation in women's health.

However, the path to equitable venture capital funding in women's health has been fraught with historical underinvestment, underscored by the stark gender disparities within the venture capital community itself. With women constituting only about 11 percent of investing partners in US venture capital firms, the dominance of male perspectives has inherently skewed funding priorities, often overlooking the significance and market potential of FemTech and women's health innovations.[186] This imbalance is starkly illustrated by the comparative funding allocated to men's health versus women's health startups; a McKinsey analysis highlighted that startups addressing erectile dysfunction secured over $1.24 billion in funding between 2019 and 2023, while those focusing on endometriosis—a condition affecting millions of women worldwide—received only $44 million.[187] Despite these challenges, the recent uptick in funding for women's health startups totaling $2.2 billion in the past four years signals a burgeoning awareness among investors of the untapped opportunities in FemTech.[188] This shift represents a financial investment and a crucial acknowledgment of the importance of women's health, marking a promising horizon for innovation and equity in healthcare.

The venture capital landscape, notorious for its competitive and often exclusionary nature, presents a unique set of challenges for female founders, particularly those spearheading startups in the women's health sector. With an astonishing 85 percent of FemTech companies being founded by women, compared to the general 15 percent across all startups, the industry not only highlights the stark gender disparities in entrepreneurship but also underscores a systemic underfunding issue that is especially pronounced in sectors led predominantly by women.[189, 190] This inherent bias is not merely a hurdle for securing financial backing; it indicates a broader, more insidious trend in venture capital that sidelines female-led innovations, especially in domains that critically address women-specific health issues. The confluence of a predominantly male investment landscape and the inherently female-centric focus of FemTech startups exacerbates this funding gap, making it an uphill battle for these enterprises to secure the necessary capital to bring transformative health solutions to market.

Yet, paradoxically, this significant challenge of underfunding female founders in women's health also carves a strategic advantage, as studies consistently show that female-led startups match and often outperform their male-led counterparts.[191] Despite receiving a fraction of the funding—2.3 percent for all-female teams and a slightly higher rate for mixed-gender teams—female entrepreneurs demonstrate remarkable efficiency, resilience, and innovation, driving their companies to achieve greater value and impact.[192] This outperformance is not limited to operational success. Still, it extends to fundraising outcomes, where female-founded ventures are shown to generate higher revenues and present better investment returns than those founded by men.[193] The discrepancy between funding levels and performance highlights a missed opportunity for investors, underscoring the need for a paradigm shift toward more equitable financing practices that recognize the inherent value and potential of female-led initiatives in women's health and beyond.

The narrative of female founders in FemTech, and more broadly in the startup ecosystem, encapsulates a broader dialogue on diversity, equity, and inclusion in venture capital. The stark underfunding of female entrepreneurs, particularly those pioneering solutions in women's health—a sector with the highest rate of female founders—illuminates the systemic barriers that women face in raising capital. However, this adversity is juxtaposed against the compelling evidence that female-founded companies are viable and often more successful and efficient than their male counterparts. The higher performance metrics of female-led startups, from lower burn rates to greater valuation growth, make a compelling case for increased investment. This duality of challenge and opportunity underscores the critical need for the venture capital industry to reevaluate its funding practices, embracing the untapped potential of female founders in FemTech and across the entrepreneurial landscape. Such a shift is not merely a matter of fairness or social equity; it is a strategic imperative for investors seeking to diversify their portfolios and capitalize on female entrepreneurs' unique insights and innovations.

We hear from various investors why they believe in FemTech as a strong investment.

## Wendy Anderson and Cristina Ljungberg, MS, MBA, Cofounders at The Case for Her

*The Case for Her is an investment portfolio geared toward issues related to menstruation, sexual wellness, and pleasure. The investors believe their investments can elevate women's health concerns and destigmatize the women's health space for other investors. Episode 106 aired April 12, 2021.*

**Why and how do you invest in women's health?**

Investing in women's health is a passion of ours and a critical need in the world today. We believe that by addressing key women's health issues, we can make a substantial impact not only on individual lives but also on societies at large. Our investment in women's health is driven by the realization that women's health issues have been historically underfunded and overlooked despite having far-reaching implications.

We invest in women's health through our philanthropic investment portfolio, The Case for Her. Our approach is unique in that we provide grant funding and make equity investments, convertible loans, and more. We're financially agnostic and focus on what will make the biggest impact. Our portfolio includes investments in product companies, tech innovations, research initiatives, and grassroots organizations.

Our work's significant focus is menstrual health, sexual health, and pleasure. These areas are particularly stigmatized and underfunded, and we can create real change by breaking the silence and taboo around these topics. Our investments range from menstrual health apps like Clue to organizations working on menstrual health in various parts of the world. We also invest in companies and projects that address sexual health and pleasure, recognizing the importance of this aspect of women's well-being.

Ultimately, our goal is to catalyze more funding for women's health. We hope to see a future where investments in women's health are not an exception but a norm, and where women's health issues receive the attention and resources they rightfully deserve.

**What is your investment thesis? What companies have you invested in and why?**

Our approach is unique in that traditional investment frameworks do not bind us. We use a mix of grant funding, equity investments, and convertible loans, tailoring our financial support to best suit the needs of the initiative or company we're supporting. This flexibility allows us to be responsive and effective in our investments.

Our portfolio is diverse in terms of the companies and projects we've invested in, spanning different geographies and approaches. For example, we've invested in Clue, a leading menstrual health app, which is a testament to our belief in the power of technology to improve women's health education and awareness. Another investment is in Sustain Natural, which provides products from menstrual care to sexual wellness, aligning with our focus on holistic women's health.

We've also supported social enterprises like B-Girl and AfriPads, which are significantly impacting the menstrual health space through innovative products and sustainable business models. These investments reflect our commitment to health outcomes, economic empowerment, and environmental sustainability.

In the realm of sexual health and pleasure, we've invested in companies like Unbound, which is pioneering in the space of sexual wellness and challenging societal norms and taboos. This aligns with our aim to normalize conversations around sexual health and pleasure and make these essential aspects of well-being more accessible.

Our investment decisions are driven by the potential for impact, the ability to fill gaps in the women's health market, and the opportunity to challenge and change the status quo. We're looking for companies and initiatives that are not just commercially viable, but also have a profound social impact, especially in stigmatized or underserved areas.

## Carolee Lee, Founder and CEO at Women's Health Access Matters (WHAM)

*Women's Health Access Matters, or WHAM, aims to accelerate women's health research through increasing awareness of inequities and closing funding gaps. Episode 211 aired May 31, 2023.*

### Why has women's health been so underfunded by the government?

Women's health has been historically underfunded due to a combination of systemic biases, lack of representation, and historical medical practices. Traditionally, the medical research community and healthcare systems have been male dominated, leading to a focus on men's health issues and an assumption that findings could be generalized to women. This gender bias in research and healthcare has resulted in a lack of understanding and appropriate treatment for women's specific health needs.

Another factor is the historical absence of women in positions of influence within the medical research community and healthcare policy-making. This gender disparity meant that women's health issues were not prioritized or adequately represented at decision-making levels. Consequently, research funding was often allocated to areas perceived as more important or universal, which typically did not include women-specific health concerns.

Moreover, there has been a long-standing misconception that women's health is limited to reproductive health, overlooking the broader spectrum of health issues that disproportionately or uniquely affect women, such as cardiovascular diseases, autoimmune disorders, and certain cancers. This narrow view has further contributed to underfunding women's health research.

Additionally, societal attitudes and stigmas around discussing women's health issues openly have played a role. For a long time, topics related to women's health, particularly reproductive and sexual health, were considered taboo, limiting public discourse and advocacy for better funding and research.

## What are the economic returns and benefits of funding women's health?

Investing in women's health research is not just a matter of social justice or ethical necessity; it's also an economic imperative with significant returns. The economic benefits of funding women's health extend far beyond the individual level, impacting society and the economy. Women control 60 percent of the wealth, are responsible for 85 percent of consumer spending decisions, and make 80 percent of healthcare decisions.

First, let's consider the workforce. Women constitute approximately half of the global workforce. When women are healthy, they are more productive, take fewer sick days, and contribute more effectively to their workplaces and economies. Poor health among women, on the other hand, leads to increased healthcare costs and decreased productivity.

For instance, the WHAM Report, which we have been heavily involved in, provides concrete figures to illustrate these benefits. The report found that an investment of $300 million (double the current funding) in researching major diseases that affect women could yield up to $13 billion in economic returns. Better health outcomes lead to reduced healthcare costs and increased productivity.

To give you specific examples, consider diseases like autoimmune disorders, heart disease, and Alzheimer's, which disproportionately affect women. We can develop more effective treatments and preventive strategies by investing more in researching these conditions. This would improve the quality of life for millions of women and reduce the economic burden of these diseases. For example, 66 percent of Alzheimer's disease patients are women, which costs the US economy billions annually in caregiving and medical expenses. (In 2020, Alzheimer's disease cost the US economy $305 billion.) Even with this in mind, just 12 percent of the $2.4 billion 2019 NIH Alzheimer's budget went to women-focused research. To break down this NIH Alzheimer's funding disparity, in practice, it equates to just $3 per woman and $24 per man. By investing in research specific to women's experiences with Alzheimer's, we can reduce these costs significantly.

Furthermore, investing in women's health research can drive innovation in the healthcare industry, leading to new medical technologies, drugs, and therapies that have broader applications beyond women's health. This can stimulate economic growth and create new markets and job opportunities.

## Carli Sapir, Founding Partner at Amboy Street Ventures

*Amboy Street Ventures focuses on investing in sexual health and women's health technology startups that are progressing in the industry in America and Europe. Episode 119 aired June 8, 2021.*

**How large is the sexual wellness market?**

The female sexual health market is part of a broader category that, when considering pleasure, women's health, and sexual health for all genders, is estimated at around $180 billion. This includes focusing on pure pleasure products and those that integrate a health aspect, which is critical to our investment thesis at Amboy Street Ventures. The reason for our specific focus on health-integrated pleasure is due to the significant, yet unaddressed, needs within this sector, especially those that cater to women and all genders inclusively.

The market is indeed growing, propelled by increasing awareness and demand for products and solutions that not only address sexual health but do so in a way that's healthy, safe, and educationally supportive. This growth is driven by a shift in societal attitudes toward more openness and acceptance of sexual wellness as an integral part of overall health and technological advancements that enable innovative product development.

I'm excited to invest in this market for several reasons. First, there's a palpable gap in solutions that genuinely cater to the nuanced needs of women and diverse genders, especially when it comes to sexual health and wellness. This gap represents both a challenge and an opportunity for startups to innovate and investors to support meaningful solutions. Furthermore, the potential for social impact is immense; by investing in this space, we're not just funding businesses but also promoting a healthier, more open society that acknowledges and addresses sexual health without stigma or taboo.

Moreover, the financial opportunity must be recognized. With menopause alone being identified as a $600 billion industry and recognizing that women account for 80 percent of health spending, the economic potential for startups that effectively address women's health and sexual wellness is significant. Our focus at Amboy Street Ventures is to bridge the capital gap, supporting startups poised to meet these burgeoning market needs with innovative, health-focused solutions.

Investing in female sexual health and wellness is more than a financial endeavor; it's a commitment to changing the narrative around sexual health, breaking down barriers, and fostering an environment where health and pleasure go hand in hand. It's about recognizing and acting on the vast potential of this market to improve lives and societies.

### What challenges do founders and investors face in the sexual wellness industry?

Raising capital for a sexual wellness fund or company presents several distinct challenges, primarily due to societal stigmas and conservative investor mindsets. The primary challenge is overcoming the hesitancy of investors who may not be comfortable with or fully understand the importance and potential of the sexual wellness sector. This discomfort stems from long-standing taboos and a lack of awareness about the significance of sexual health as part of overall well-being. Consequently, these factors can lead to a scarcity of capital available to founders in this space, despite the clear demand and market opportunity.

Another challenge is the difficulty in conveying the scale of the market opportunity to investors who may not be part of the target demographic or may not recognize the comprehensive needs within sexual wellness. The perception of sexual wellness as a niche or controversial area rather than a critical aspect of healthcare and lifestyle further complicates fundraising efforts.

To overcome these challenges, it's essential to educate potential investors about the market's size, growth potential, and the societal impact of investing in sexual wellness. This includes presenting hard data, market research, and consumer trends highlighting demand and financial opportunity. Building a compelling narrative around the positive social impact of these investments, such as promoting sexual health, education, and inclusivity, can also help align with investors' values and interests.

Personal challenges I've faced include navigating investor discomfort and the need to advocate for the importance of this space continually. To overcome these, I've focused on building a strong network of like-minded investors and founders who share a vision for the potential of sexual wellness. By coinvesting with partners who understand the market and leveraging our collective expertise, we've created a more compelling case for investment. Additionally, showcasing successful case studies and returns from the sector helps demonstrate its viability and profitability, gradually changing perceptions and opening more doors for funding.

## Maurissa Bell, CPA, CA, Private Equity Investor

*Partnering with entrepreneurs at a top-decile private equity fund with $4+ billion assets under management to help build strategically significant businesses across various industries.*
*Episode 197 aired February 22, 2023.*

### What opportunity do you see in women's health for private equity?

The opportunity in women's health is expansive and profoundly impactful, reflecting a sector ripe for innovation and growth. Women represent approximately 50 percent of the global population, yet the healthcare sector has historically underserved and overlooked their specific needs. The recent surge in attention and investment in women's health, or FemTech, signifies a pivotal shift toward rectifying this imbalance.

The most compelling aspects of the women's health sector are its nascent state and immense potential due to women having children later in life, driving a higher need for services, and women making more money than they ever have in history. Despite being a fundamental aspect of healthcare, women's health has only recently begun to attract the significant attention it deserves from investors, innovators, and healthcare providers alike. This delayed focus presents a unique opportunity for growth and innovation, making it an attractive arena for private equity investment.

Private equity involves investing in companies that are not publicly traded on a stock exchange. Private equity fund managers often seek to generate returns by enhancing the performance of the companies they invest in over the course of a holding period. There are various types of private investment strategies which typically invest in more mature companies in contrast to venture capital which invests in startups.

Significant deals in the past few years underscore this sector's burgeoning interest and confidence. For instance, KKR, a global alternative asset manager focused on private equity, acquired IVI RMA, a fertility clinic, for €3 billion. EQT, a leading private equity firm, purchased

Igenomix, another global IVF clinic, which was later sold to Vitrolife for an enterprise value of €1.25 billion. These highlight the global fertility market's growth and investment potential. These transactions are not isolated events but a broader trend of increasing investment and consolidation in women's health, particularly in fertility clinics and related services.

The fertility market, in particular, demonstrates the high demand and potential for returns in women's health. Despite advancements, there's a recognized need for more data-driven solutions, especially in improving fertility treatments' success rates. AI and innovative technologies present opportunities to enhance these outcomes, indicating a substantial growth area that aligns with private equity's investment thesis of supporting companies that benefit from technological advancements and market growth.

Moreover, the demographics and societal shifts underscore the potential in the menopause market, reflecting another key area for innovation and investment. An aging population and increased recognition of menopause's impact on productivity and health highlight the need for solutions catering to this stage of women's health. The alignment of economic incentives, such as the potential to mitigate productivity losses in the workforce, further validates the investment thesis in this space.

Private equity's interest in women's health stems from the sector's potential for high growth, the significant impact on a substantial portion of the population, and the opportunity to drive meaningful improvements in healthcare outcomes. By investing in women's health, private equity can be crucial in accelerating innovation, improving access to care, and addressing long-standing gaps in healthcare delivery.

## How has private equity historically thought about women's health? What advice do you have for founders considering private equity investment?

The history of private equity's involvement in women's health has been relatively recent but rapidly evolving. Historically, the broader healthcare sector attracted private equity due to its resilience and growth potential, but women's health specifically was often overlooked. This oversight is not due to a lack of opportunity or need but rather a historical undervaluation of women-specific healthcare needs and opportunities. In recent years, however, we've seen a paradigm shift. High-profile investments underscore a growing recognition of the value and potential within the women's health sector. This change is driven by a combination of factors, including increased demand for women-specific healthcare services, a growing FemTech market, and a broader societal push toward gender equity in healthcare.

Looking forward, I anticipate private equity will play a pivotal role in shaping the future of women's health. The sector's strong industry fundamentals and significant growth potential present a compelling investment thesis for private equity firms. We will likely see increased investment in fertility, menopause management, and digital health solutions catering specifically to women. This will drive innovation and improve access and outcomes for women's healthcare services. Furthermore, as the sector matures, private equity can support scaling operations, navigating regulatory environments, and fostering strategic partnerships, accelerating growth and innovation in women's health.

My advice for companies considering private equity investment centers on preparation, clarity, and alignment. First, understand your deal priorities. Know what you're looking for in a partnership or investment, whether a full sale, a majority stake, or a minority investment, and what you plan to achieve with the investment (secondary sell down, recapitalization of balance sheet, growth equity, etc.). Your growth strategy should be clear and compelling, illustrating your vision for the company and how additional capital will help you achieve it.

Second, prepare your business for scrutiny. Ensure your financials are in order, understand your market position, and be ready to present a well-articulated plan for growth. This preparation will not only aid in attracting the right investment partner but also secure favorable terms.

Last, seek alignment with your investment partner where the full company is not sold (buyout). The relationship between a company and its private equity investors is profoundly collaborative. It's crucial to partner with a firm that provides capital and aligns with your vision, values, and growth aspirations. Ask about the fund's strategy, its sources of capital, and its approach during challenging times, and request references from their portfolio companies. Knowing who you're joining a business with is paramount to a successful partnership.

## Jessica Karr, MS, MBA, Founder and Managing Director at Coyote Ventures

*The firm focuses on seed-stage investments and considers companies innovating in conditions that solely, differently, and disproportionally affect women's health. Episode Bonus 10 aired June 25, 2021.*

### What is Coyote Ventures's investment thesis?

Coyote Ventures invests in early stage companies innovating in women's health and wellness. Our fund is $10 million, and we focus primarily on seed-stage companies, aiming to be the partner that helps these companies bridge the gap from seed to Series A funding. While we primarily invest at the seed stage, we're also open to supporting companies outside of this stage if they align with our mission and demonstrate exceptional potential.

Our investment thesis is grounded in the belief that every area of FemTech is underserved yet brimming with opportunity for significant impact. We are particularly drawn to science-driven products that can make a real difference in women's lives. Our interests span biotech, consumer products, apps, diagnostics, and digital health, reflecting the diverse needs and challenges within women's health. However, we've chosen to steer clear of highly regulated spaces like therapeutics and medical devices, as these require specialized expertise and approaches that differ from our investment focus.

The excitement about investing in women's health stems from the sheer magnitude of unaddressed needs and the potential for transformative impact. Consider that one in four women will experience an abortion in their lifetime, yet only a handful of startups address this need. The disparity between the prevalence of women's health issues and the solutions available is staggering, presenting a ripe opportunity for innovation and investment. By supporting companies that address these underserved areas, we're not just funding businesses; we're championing gender equality and empowering women to demand better and more holistic solutions in their lives.

What truly excites me about this space is its intersection with gender equality and dismantling systemic barriers to women's health. Investing in FemTech is an opportunity to catalyze change on a fundamental level, breaking down stigmas and fostering a world where women's health is prioritized and well-understood. Through Coyote Ventures, we're building a portfolio that promises significant returns and contributes to a more equitable and healthy future for women everywhere.

**How is Coyote Ventures different from traditional venture funds?**

Coyote Ventures differentiates itself by deeply focusing on women's health and wellness, investing not just financially but with a comprehensive understanding and passion for the sector. Our commitment to seed-stage companies in this underserved area, combined with our specific knowledge and network, positions us uniquely to support founders as investors and true partners.

Our fund is distinct in its approach to startup relationships and wellness. Recognizing the unique challenges women and underrepresented founders face, we emphasize a healthy balance, supporting not only their companies' growth but also their personal well-being. This includes the novel idea of hosting founder retreats to foster community, inspiration, and holistic well-being, acknowledging that great work often comes from a place of health and balance, not a relentless grind.

This model speaks to the emergence of a new investor and venture capitalist type, one that values diversity, equity, and the importance of nurturing founder well-being alongside business metrics. We represent a shift toward more empathetic, informed, and socially conscious investment practices, focusing on creating meaningful impact alongside financial returns. As part of this new wave, we're challenging traditional venture capital norms and paving the way for a more inclusive and supportive venture ecosystem.

## Lu Zhang, MS, Founder and Managing Partner at Fusion Fund

*Fusion Fund supports early stage entrepreneurs looking to build globally disruptive companies using innovative technologies to drive systemic change. Episode 185 aired October 31, 2022.*

**What is the role of women in funding women's health companies?**

Female leadership in finance is pivotal in funding FemTech for several reasons. First, women leaders bring essential perspectives and understanding of women's health issues, which are often overlooked or underrepresented in the male-dominated finance sector. This insight is crucial for recognizing the value and potential of FemTech startups, driving more informed and empathetic investment decisions.

Second, female finance leaders can influence investment priorities and strategies within their organizations, advocating for a more significant allocation of resources to FemTech. By doing so, they address the historical funding gap that FemTech companies face, helping to bring innovative women's health solutions to market faster.

Additionally, female financial leaders serve as role models and mentors for women entrepreneurs, providing guidance, support, and access to critical fundraising and business development networks. This mentorship is invaluable for navigating the challenges of raising capital, particularly in a field that requires investors to understand complex healthcare and technological issues.

Furthermore, female leadership in finance contributes to creating a more inclusive investment ecosystem that values diversity and innovation. By supporting FemTech, these leaders are not just investing in women's health but also advocating for gender equity in healthcare and technology, driving systemic change.

**Tell us about the business models you see in women's health startups.**

Women's health companies often adopt a direct-to-consumer (DTC) business model, leveraging digital platforms to reach their audience directly. This model enables personalized engagement and education about women's health issues, fostering a community around their solutions. While effective, the DTC approach primarily targets consumers already seeking solutions, potentially limiting its reach to those unaware of their needs or available innovations.

Another prevalent model is selling to businesses (B2B), where FemTech companies partner with healthcare providers, employers, or insurance companies to integrate their solutions into existing healthcare frameworks. This approach facilitates broader adoption and reimbursement pathways but requires navigating complex sales cycles and regulatory landscapes.

Looking forward, I advocate for innovative business models that bridge the gap between DTC and B2B, fostering collaborations that bring FemTech solutions to a wider audience while ensuring sustainability and scalability. Specifically, I see immense potential in models that engage insurance companies and healthcare providers as channels and active partners in promoting women's health innovation. This could include value-based care models, where payments are tied to the efficacy of FemTech solutions in improving patient outcomes, encouraging the adoption of technologies that genuinely make a difference.

Moreover, I am keen on seeing FemTech companies explore public-private partnerships, leveraging governmental support to address public health challenges related to women's health. Such models can significantly impact underfunded areas like maternal health, reproductive health, and conditions disproportionately affecting women, such as autoimmune diseases.

## Faz Bashi, MD, Lead Venture Investor at Portfolia FemTech Funds I, II, and III

*Dr. Faz Bashi is the lead investor at the Portfolia FemTech Funds I, II, and III, which invest in female health and wellness startups. Portfolia creates investment funds focused on markets that women drive, such as women's health, active aging, consumer, enterprise, fashion, tech, and beauty. Episode 28 aired July 15, 2020.*

**How has the female health investment landscape changed?**

The female health investment landscape has undergone a significant transformation, moving from a narrow focus on specific areas like UTIs and organic tampons to recognizing the vast expanse of women's health needs. This shift underscores a growing awareness among investors that women's health encompasses a wide range of conditions and challenges, many of which have been historically underserved and overlooked.

Areas of strategic investment now increasingly include conditions like endometriosis and pelvic pain, conditions that affect a significant portion of the female population yet have seen comparatively little innovation or investment. The focus is also expanding to include complex health issues such as fibromyalgia and specific types of cancer that disproportionately affect women. These areas represent a pressing health need and a substantial market opportunity that has yet to be fully tapped.

Statistics and success stories underscore the potential for significant returns on investment in female health. For instance, Boston Scientific's acquisition of nVision Medical for $275 million in April 2018 highlights the economic viability of investing in FemTech. It indicates that there is real financial value to be unlocked in addressing the health needs of half the world's population.

Furthermore, Maven Health's $45 million funding round is a testament to the growing interest and confidence in FemTech's potential. This, alongside other emerging success stories, serves as a beacon for current and potential investors, signaling the fertile ground for innovation and economic gain within the sector.

However, the landscape is not without its challenges. Despite these advancements, there is still a need for a broader acknowledgment and deeper understanding of the comprehensive nature of women's health needs. Investing in FemTech requires a willingness to explore beyond the surface and to seek out and support innovations that tackle the more complex, less visible issues affecting women's health.

**What advice do you have for founders and investors in FemTech?**

For investors interested in FemTech, I advise recognizing the enormity and diversity of the opportunity that lies within women's health. The landscape is shifting, with more sophisticated and complex challenges being addressed by today's entrepreneurs. Investors should seek to understand the specific conditions and areas within FemTech that are underserved and represent significant market opportunities. Look for companies that are not just innovating for innovation but are solving real problems that affect a substantial portion of the population. The economic potential in FemTech is significant, as evidenced by successful acquisitions and funding rounds. Do your homework, understand the science, the market, and, importantly, the impact of these solutions on women's lives.

For FemTech founders, my counsel is to focus on the areas within women's health that are still ripe for innovation. Conditions like endometriosis, pelvic pain, and fibromyalgia are just the tip of the iceberg. It's imperative to build solutions that are not only clinically effective but also economically viable. Understand your market deeply, know your user's pain points, and build with empathy. Forge strong relationships with investors who provide capital and value and understand the FemTech space. Remember, mentorship is a shortcut to success; seek advisers who can guide and challenge you and open doors for you.

The FemTech industry, to be successful, needs a cohesive ecosystem that supports innovation at every stage. This includes financial investment, mentorship, access to clinical trials, and a supportive regulatory environment. Success stories must be highlighted and learned from, creating a cycle of inspiration and aspiration for current and future founders. The industry needs more champions within the investment community willing to bet on FemTech, recognizing its potential to change lives and generate economic returns. Collaboration between startups, investors, healthcare providers, and regulatory bodies is crucial. Last, the industry must continue to elevate the conversation around women's health, advocating for the importance and necessity of innovation in this space.

FemTech's success hinges on the ability to address complex health challenges with innovative, effective solutions that meet the needs of women globally. This requires passion, resilience, and a deep understanding of the healthcare and business aspects of bringing new solutions to market.

## Cheryl Campos, MBA, Former Head of Venture Growth and Partnerships at Republic

*Republic is a private crowdfunding investing platform where accredited and nonaccredited individuals can invest in private startups in exchange for equity. Episode 130 aired August 23, 2021.*

### What challenges do FemTech companies face when fundraising from venture capital?

FemTech companies face several notable challenges when fundraising from venture capitalists, largely due to systemic issues within the investment community and societal perceptions of women's health. One significant challenge is the lack of awareness and understanding from predominantly male investors who may not personally relate to the problems FemTech ventures are solving. This gap in personal experience can lead to a lack of interest or perceived value in FemTech innovations, as highlighted by the anecdote involving sex tech companies facing biases due to the nature of their products. Such instances underscore a broader issue: the struggle for recognition and acceptance within technological and investment spaces that traditionally prioritize more universally applicable or lucrative sectors.

Another challenge stems from the historical underrepresentation of women in venture capital (VC) and investment decision-making. With women significantly underrepresented in these positions, FemTech companies often pitch to individuals who may need a direct connection to or understanding of the health issues being addressed. This disconnect can result in FemTech ventures being perceived as niche or limited in potential, even though women's health issues impact half of the global population. The underfunding of FemTech startups is a manifestation of broader gender disparities in venture funding, where despite women representing a substantial portion of the consumer market and healthcare decision-makers, ventures led by women or targeting women's health issues receive a fraction of available venture capital.

Compounding these challenges is the issue of predatory capital, where FemTech founders, in desperate need of funding, may accept unfavorable terms that disproportionately benefit the investor at the expense of the company's long-term success. This situation is exacerbated by a lack of alternative funding sources that understand and value the FemTech space, further hindering these companies' growth and innovation potential.

The solution to these challenges lies in increasing the representation of women in VC, educating investors on the value and necessity of FemTech solutions, and developing funding mechanisms that recognize and support the unique needs and potential of FemTech ventures. Equity crowdfunding platforms like Republic, which offer a more democratized approach to investing, present one avenue for FemTech companies to bypass traditional VC barriers and access capital from a broader, potentially more empathetic, supportive investor base.

## What is equity crowdfunding? How has it been uniquely useful to FemTech startups?

Equity crowdfunding is raising capital that allows companies to source investments from a broad public audience, not just accredited investors or venture capitalists. This approach democratizes investment, enabling individuals to invest small amounts of money in startups or growing businesses in exchange for equity. It leverages the power of the crowd, utilizing online platforms to aggregate numerous small investments to reach the company's funding goal.

For FemTech companies, equity crowdfunding presents a unique opportunity to overcome some traditional barriers they face in venture capital fundraising. Given that the FemTech sector often deals with issues that are either overlooked or undervalued by traditional investment communities, largely due to a lack of personal connection or understanding, crowdfunding allows these companies to appeal directly to the public. This enables them to raise necessary funds and build a community of supporters and potential customers who are invested in their success, both financially and emotionally. FemTech ventures can leverage the collective support of individuals who understand and value their products and services, bypassing the need for approval from a few gatekeepers in the venture capital world.

Successful examples of FemTech companies that have utilized crowdfunding to raise funds highlight the potential of this approach. Dame Products, a company focusing on sexual wellness and education, is a notable example. They've successfully raised funds through crowdfunding, showcasing the ability of FemTech companies to attract significant public support and investment. This success story, among others, illustrates the viability of equity crowdfunding as an alternative funding route for FemTech ventures, enabling them to capitalize on public interest and support to scale their operations and impact.

Equity crowdfunding provides the capital FemTech companies' need to grow and offers a platform for raising awareness and fostering community engagement around women's health issues. It's a powerful tool that aligns financial goals with broader missions to improve women's lives and health outcomes globally.

## Maria D. Toler, MBA, Founding Partner at Steelsky Ventures

*Steelsky Ventures invests in companies that improve access, care, and outcomes in women's health. They invest across the spectrum of women's health in consumer health, digital health, and healthcare infrastructure. Episode 134 aired September 20, 2021.*

### What role does diversity play in FemTech entrepreneurship and investing?

Diversity among FemTech founders and investors is not just important, it's essential for creating equitable and effective healthcare solutions for all women. The reason is straightforward: Diverse teams bring a wide range of perspectives, experiences, and insights, ensuring that the products and services developed truly meet the varied needs of women from different backgrounds, cultures, and life stages. This is critical for improving women's health across the board because, historically, the healthcare system has not adequately served minority populations, including women of color.

One glaring example is the maternal mortality rate for Black and Hispanic women, which is three to four times higher overall than for White women. In certain areas, like New Jersey, it's seven times more likely, and in New York, you're ten times more likely to die if you're a Black woman giving birth. These statistics are not just numbers; they are a call to action. They highlight the dire need for innovations that cater to the specific health challenges faced by these populations.

Furthermore, considering that 42 percent of women having babies are on Medicaid, it becomes evident that we need to innovate for all tiers of the socioeconomic spectrum, not just the commercially insured. This approach fosters inclusivity and amplifies the impact FemTech can have on society by addressing underserved or previously ignored health issues.

In addition, the global perspective of FemTech innovation demonstrates that effective solutions often come from those who experience the problems firsthand. For instance, innovations emerging from regions like Africa and India are tailored to their local contexts, proving that understanding the consumer is key to developing impactful products and services. Therefore, having a woman on the team, especially in leadership positions, is not just beneficial but, in many cases, crucial for the success of FemTech companies.

### What trends and opportunities do you see in FemTech?

In FemTech, we're witnessing a saturation in certain areas, like period and fertility-tracking apps, suggesting that new entrants should look toward untapped markets for innovation. There's a clear opportunity to address the needs of menopausal women—a segment historically overlooked despite its significant potential for impact. This stage in a woman's life is ripe for innovation, from symptom management to overall well-being, highlighting a gap in the market waiting to be filled.

Another critical area is maternal mental health. With one-third of women experiencing postpartum depression, the need for accessible and effective solutions has never been more urgent. The opportunity here lies in creating innovative approaches to support women through not only postpartum depression but also the broader spectrum of mental health challenges associated with motherhood.

Globally, FemTech innovation is not confined to one region. Countries like Israel are leading in IVF and medical device innovations, while startups in Africa and India are creating solutions tailored to their unique societal and environmental contexts. This global innovation landscape underscores the vast potential for FemTech to adapt and address women's health issues across different cultures and societies.

Moreover, the spotlight on period poverty and the need for sustainable menstrual products in underprivileged areas presents an opportunity for FemTech companies to make a tangible difference. Initiatives that provide sustainable solutions, such as period underwear, can revolutionize how menstrual health is managed globally, particularly in period deserts.

In essence, FemTech is at a crossroads of opportunity, with the potential to dive deeper into underserved areas of women's health. By focusing on inclusive and diverse solutions that span from menopause to maternal mental health, FemTech can continue to be a powerful force for positive change in the healthcare landscape.

* * *

As we navigate the complex landscape of funding women's health, it becomes increasingly clear that a holistic and strategic infusion of capital is essential for fostering innovation and ensuring equitable access to healthcare for all women. The burgeoning field of FemTech, often viewed through a narrow lens, represents an expansive opportunity to address critical health needs and drive substantial economic growth. This sector, ripe for disruption, requires a multifaceted approach to funding that encompasses traditional venture capital, enlightened angel investments, progressive government grants, and visionary private equity. Each funding stream must be mobilized to champion the untapped potential within women's health, encouraging a paradigm shift that both values and invests in female-centric healthcare solutions as a priority, not an afterthought. By doing so, we can catalyze a new era of healthcare innovation that not only uplifts women but also sets a new standard for inclusivity and effectiveness in healthcare funding, ultimately leading to a healthier, more equitable future.

# Conclusion

**FEMTECH, AN INDUSTRY PIONEERED AND PROPELLED BY WOMEN,** showcases the transformative power of female leadership. Characterized by a spirit of collaboration and partnership, FemTech thrives on collective success and accountability, creating a nurturing ecosystem where toxic patriarchy is not just absent—it's irrelevant. Instead, our energies converge on dismantling systemic biases in investment, science, and healthcare, challenging the status quo not in isolation but in unity. This inclusive and progressive dynamic magnetizes more women to be drawn to the empowering and supportive environment. It's a testament to what industries can achieve when women lead and men are supportive allies and contributors, embodying the principles of equality, innovation, and mutual respect, and paving the way for a more equitable future in technology and beyond.

Recognizing and addressing the diverse needs of women from every part of the globe is paramount. The solutions that resonate with White, affluent women in the United States might not even scratch the surface of what's necessary for a Filipino woman living on a remote island. Our approach must be inclusive, harnessing innovation to cater not just to women in high-income countries but also those in low- and middle-income countries (LMICs). It's crucial to challenge the assumption that innovation flows from the wealthier nations to the LMICs; often, the reality is beautifully inverse. Consider the practice prevalent among women in LMICs of keeping their babies close, wrapped tightly against their bodies as they go about their daily tasks. This tradition sparked curiosity among researchers who replicated this method with American mothers. The findings were striking—a significant decrease in postpartum depression among those who embraced this practice. This insight stands as a powerful testament to the fact that LMICs hold invaluable wisdom, practices, and solutions from which the entire world can benefit. Embracing global diversity in women's needs and experiences is not just an act of inclusion but a strategy for uncovering universally beneficial innovations in women's health.

Despite the wealth of innovation and solutions chronicled within the pages of this book, the domain of women's health remains a vast expanse ripe for further exploration and development. Take, for instance, the prevalence of ovarian cysts, a condition that affects over 75 percent of women at some point in their lives. Astonishingly, this widespread issue has not been the beneficiary of NIH research funding, nor has it been the focus of significant scientific inquiry into ovarian cyst biology. The lack of therapeutic interventions or medical devices designed to prevent ovarian cysts highlights a glaring oversight in women's health research, often dismissed with the broad-stroke prescription of birth control as a panacea. Yet, what of the women for whom hormonal contraceptives are not an option or those who choose to avoid them? A therapeutic that enables women to ovulate while preventing the formation of a cyst will be a multibillion-dollar drug since women question being on hormonal birth control for decades at a time.

Equally pressing is the need to address women's rectal health, arguably the most stigmatized aspect of female physiology. The silence and shame surrounding discussions of women's bowel movements obscure the significant rectal health challenges many face. For example, up to 85 percent of pregnant women suffer from anal hemorrhoids, a condition starkly underserved by the current market of healthcare solutions.[194] There are numerous urinary incontinence solutions in development and thought leadership panels speaking on pelvic floor health. Yet, we rarely hear about fecal incontinence, which affects one in four women at some point in their lives. Moreover, menstrual diarrhea, affecting 28 percent of menstruating individuals, exemplifies the interconnectedness of women's reproductive and digestive health, yet remains largely unaddressed.[195] These examples represent just the tip of the iceberg in the myriad health issues facing women which demand not only destigmatization but also dedicated research, innovation, and solution development.

The path forward requires breaking the silence on these topics, encouraging open dialogue, and committing to the research and development of targeted treatments and solutions. The future of women's health is a horizon filled with untapped potential, where the last frontiers of stigma can be dismantled, and comprehensive, inclusive healthcare can emerge.

In the near future, the FemTech industry is poised for transformative growth and change, ushering in an era where women's health is not just a niche market but a forefront of medical innovation and investment. We are on the cusp of witnessing FemTech companies scaling to rival giants like Hologic, Cooper Surgical, and Procter & Gamble, diversifying the landscape of acquirers in women's health. This expansion will pave the way for significant exits and rewarding returns to investors, further fueling the industry's upward trajectory. A unique cycle of reinvestment is set to emerge, with successful FemTech founders channeling their insights and capital back into the sector, creating a robust, self-sustaining ecosystem dedicated to advancing women's health.

As the industry matures, we will see a strategic shift away from the saturation of products in fertility and menstruation toward uncharted territories of women's health, driven by a deeper understanding of biological research, drug targets, and disease mechanisms. The entry of more men into FemTech will bring additional perspectives, although the heart of the industry will continue to be led by women, especially in research and development roles. An increase in dedicated laboratories and the formation of new venture funds focused on FemTech will amplify scientific discoveries and unprecedented funding for women's health. Coupled with a destigmatization of women's health issues, we're going to witness a societal shift where conversations about menstruation, breastfeeding, contraception, and menopause are normalized in public and mainstream media. This openness will not only foster innovation but also promote a more inclusive and understanding healthcare environment for women globally.

As the FemTech movement continues to gain momentum, it's inevitable that we'll encounter resistance. This backlash is a common reaction to societal shifts, especially those aimed at empowering historically underrepresented groups. The recent overturning of abortion rights in the United States serves as a stark reminder of the challenges facing the advancement of women's health. However, it's crucial that we remain focused on our primary goal: to ensure that sex and gender are recognized as critical biological variables in science, healthcare, and innovation.

While healthtech encompasses both male and female health solutions, the glaring disparities in solutions specifically designed for women highlight the existing gap that FemTech seeks to fill. This new focus may initially create discomfort and resistance from different generations and geographies, particularly those with entrenched patriarchal views and societal norms surrounding women's health. Yet, it's important to remember that systemic change is a gradual process. As cultural perceptions evolve, what is considered normal or taboo will transform, paving the way for more inclusive and comprehensive healthcare solutions. The resistance we face today will eventually give way to a new understanding and acceptance of women's health needs, marking a significant step forward in the journey toward equity in healthcare. Just as the generations of women before us fought for the right to education, voting, and financial independence (without a husband to cosign), we will fight and eventually gain our right to equal healthcare solutions. Ironically, have we not witnessed how providing women with more liberties inevitably benefits everyone? Optimizing women's health and wellness to be on par with men's will bolster the health and wellness of every gender, sex, and age.

As we navigate the complexities of today's world, the foundation we're laying in understanding female biology is crucial, not only for the immediate future but also for addressing global challenges on the horizon. Two significant issues stand out due to their far-reaching implications: the worldwide decline in fertility rates amid alarming overpopulation concerns and the advent of human space exploration. These topics, seemingly distinct, share a common thread in their reliance on FemTech advancements to guide equitable and informed decisions.

The first challenge involves the paradox of decreasing fertility rates against the backdrop of Earth's overpopulation. This dichotomy is beginning to spark global debates centered on who should be aided in conceiving and who should limit their offspring—a discussion fraught with potential for deep-seated racism, economic disparities, and ethical dilemmas. High-income countries may face declining populations with adverse economic impacts, as seen in China's shift from its one-child policy to encouraging larger families. This governmental influence on women's reproductive rights highlights the critical need for FemTech in shaping policies that balance sustainability with economic needs, ensuring women's autonomy over their bodies is respected in the discourse on global population management.

Equally pressing is the consideration of female biology in the burgeoning field of space exploration. With women representing a small fraction of astronauts (11 percent) and spacewalk participants (6.6 percent; fifteen of the 225 recorded to date), it's clear that gender-specific research in space science is lacking.[196] From understanding menstruation in zero gravity to ensuring space suits fit female astronauts, FemTech has a pivotal role to play. NASA has admittedly come a long way since 1983 when engineers planned to send Sally Ride for a one-week trip into space with one-hundred tampons. But as recently as 2019 a historic all-female spacewalk was canceled due to a lack of female space suits.[197] Recent findings on women's heightened sensitivity to space radiation further underscore the necessity for targeted research and solutions. As humanity stands on the cusp of colonizing Mars and mining the moon, ensuring female health is prioritized will be crucial for the success and well-being of all spacefarers.

These imminent challenges underscore the indispensable role of FemTech in not only advancing women's health on Earth but also in preparing humanity for life beyond our planet. By focusing on FemTech today, we are investing in a future where decisions regarding population management and space exploration are informed by comprehensive understanding and respect for female biology. This is not merely a step forward for women's health; it's a leap toward a more equitable and sustainable future for all of humanity.

As we reflect on the FemTech industry's trajectory and the contents of this book, it's vital to acknowledge the ongoing debate around whether FemTech should simply be classified under healthtech. But one may argue that healthtech is in fact "mentech" considering that our current healthcare system is deeply rooted in a male-centric scientific understanding of health. Alas, my aspiration is, however, for FemTech to eventually merge and be synonymous with healthtech, reflecting a healthcare education system where menstruation and menopause are taught with the same emphasis as viral infections and obesity. While FemTech, like obstetrics and gynecology, provides a crucial platform for female-specific health discussions, the ultimate goal is for all healthcare professionals to incorporate sex and gender considerations across all medical disciplines, breaking free from silos while still cherishing our dedicated space for female health discussions.

The hope that this book, in time, becomes outdated is a testament to the rapid pace at which FemTech and women's health are evolving. Significant milestones in women's health have been made during the writing of this manuscript, such as the constitutional right to abortion in France, FDA approval of the first over-the-counter birth control in the US, novel therapeutics for menopausal hot flashes, and the identification of the protein causing morning sickness, all signifying tremendous progress. These developments, alongside the creation of a dedicated White House task force for women's health with $100 million dedicated to women's health research, underscore the dynamism and potential for even greater achievements in FemTech. This book aims to serve not only as a contemporary resource but also as a historical case study, illustrating the transformative power of inclusion and representation in STEM and innovation, inspiring future movements toward equity in other underserved communities.

At its core, enhancing women's health transcends the boundaries of healthcare; it's fundamentally about fostering women's equality. Healthy women have the foundation to achieve financial independence, actively participate in the workforce, and drive innovation and discovery. It empowers us to occupy seats at decision-making tables, lead with authority, and initiate substantial societal change. The progress women have made, even amid health challenges, is remarkable. Imagine the bounds of what can be achieved when we are not just surviving but thriving. The journey toward women's health and, by extension, women's equality, is not just a pursuit of wellness—it's a pathway to unlocking the untapped potential of half the world's population. In fostering a world where women's health is prioritized, we pave the way for a future where female equality is not an aspiration but a reality, demonstrating what is truly possible when we are well.

# Take Action

The interviews featured in this book were all taken from the *FemTech Focus* podcast. To hear the full interviews and gain even more insights, listen to the show on your favorite streaming platform. You'll find over one hundred additional interviews not included here. Additionally, I, the author, have created a special series of episodes with behind-the-scenes stories and product spotlights for each of the sixteen chapters of this book.

Support these FemTech innovators by investing in their crowdfunding campaigns, donating to their foundations, purchasing their products for yourself or loved ones, and asking your healthcare providers if they have heard of and intend to adopt these solutions. Share what you've learned from this book with people in your life, both men and women, young and old. The more we discuss women's challenges and the solutions that exist, the less stigma will persist. Making women's health mainstream benefits us all. Additionally, women's health is uniquely influenced by policy in academics and the government at all levels. I beseech you, support leaders and laws that benefit women, female, and girl's health.

This is not just a book. It's a movement, and you're now a part of it. Together, we can unlock a better future for women's health.

# List of Figures

# Appendix: Company List

**List of companies and guests featured in this book in alphabetical order by company name:**

# Endnotes

## Introduction

1 National Institutes of Health. "NIH Inclusion Outreach Toolkit: How to Engage, Recruit, and Retain Women in Clinical Research." https://orwh.od.nih.gov/toolkit/recruitment/history#1.

2 Temkin, Sarah M., Samia Noursi, Judith G. Regensteiner, Pamela Stratton, and Janine A. Clayton. 2017. "Perspectives From Advancing National Institutes of Health Research to Inform and Improve the Health of Women: A Conference Summary." *Obstetrics & Gynecology* 140, no. 1: 10-19. https://doi.org/10.1097/AOG.0000000000004821.

3 Kim, Jun Yeob, Kyoungmi Min, Hee Young Paik, and Suk Kyeong Lee. 2021. "Sex omission and male bias are still widespread in cell experiments." *American Journal of Physiology: Cell Physiology* 320, no. 5: C742–C749 https://doi.org/10.1152/ajpcell.00358.2020.

4 Ellingrud, Kweilin, Lucy Pérez, Anouk Petersen, and Valentina Sartori. 2024. *Closing the Women's Health Gap: A $1 Trillion Opportunity to Improve Lives and Economies*, World Economic Forum. https://www.weforum.org/publications/closing-the-women-s-health-gap-a-1-trillion-opportunity-to-improve-lives-and-economies/.

5 Faculty of Health and Medical Sciences. 2019. "Across Diseases, Women Are Diagnosed Later Than Men." University of Copenhagen. March 10, 2019. https://www.cpr.ku.dk/cpr-news/2019/study-across-diseases-women-are-diagnosed-later-than-men.

6 Westwood, Shannon, Mackenzie Fannin, Fadumo Ali, Justice Thigpen, Rachel Tatro, Amanda Hernandez, Cadynce Peltzer, Mariah Hildebrand, Alexnys Fernandez-Pacheco, Jonathan R. Raymond-Lezman, and Robin J. Jacobs. 2023. "Disparities in Women With Endometriosis Regarding Access to Care, Diagnosis, Treatment, and Management in the United States: A Scoping Review." *Cureus* 15, no. 5: e38765 (May 9, 2023). https://doi.org/10.7759/cureus.38765.

7 Barreto, Brittany, Megan Fuller, Ariella Tal, Saumya Bhatia, Jennifer Ma, Disha Trivedi, Cristy Gross, Anna-Maria Strasser, and Alexandria Farmer. 2024. *2023 FemTech Landscape Report*, FemHealth Insights. https://www.femhealthinsights.com/reports/p/2023-femtech-landscape-report.

8 Barreto, *Landscape Report.*

9 Barreto, *Landscape Report.*

10 Barreto, *Landscape Report.*

11 Koning, Rembrand, Sampsa Samila, and John-Paul Ferguson. 2021. "Who do we invent for? Patents by women focus more on women's health, but few women get to invent." *American Association for the Advancement of Science* 372, no. 6548: 1345–1348. https://doi.org/10.1126/science.aba6990.

12 National Center for Science and Engineering Statistics (NCSES). 2023. *Diversity and STEM: Women, Minorities, and Persons with Disabilities*, National Center for Science and Engineering Statistics. https://ncses.nsf.gov/wmpd.

13 Kali Pal, Kusum, Ricky Li, Kim Piaget, Silja Baller, and Saadia Zahidi. 2023. *Global Gender Gap Report 2023*, World Economic Forum. https://www.weforum.org/publications/global-gender-gap-report-2023/.

14 Stengel, Geri. 2022. "Women Angel Investors: A Movement That Has Taken Off." Forbes. August 3, 2022. https://www.forbes.com/sites/geristengel/2022/08/03/women-angel-investors-a-movement-that-has-taken-off/.

15 Barreto, *Landscape Report.*

## Chapter 1

16 Bellofiore, Nadia, Stacey J. Ellery, Jared Mamrot, David W. Walker, Peter Temple-Smith, and Hayley Dickinson. 2017. "First evidence of a menstruating rodent: the spiny mouse (*Acomys cahirinus*)." *American Journal of Obstetrics and Gynecology* 216, no. 1: 40.e1-40.e11. https://doi.org/10.1016/j.ajog.2016.07.041.

17 Al-Hafez, Leen, and Heather Fisher. 2023. "Can genetic testing explain the cause of recurrent miscarriages?" *UT Southwestern Medical Center*, September 19, 2023. https://utswmed.org/medblog/miscarriage-genetics/.

18 United Nations Children's Fund. 2018. "Fast Facts: Nine things you didn't know about menstruation." May 25, 2028. https://www.unicef.org/press-releases/fast-facts-nine-things-you-didnt-know-about-menstruation.

19 Fortune Business Insights. 2024. "Feminine Hygiene Products Market Size, Share, & Industry Analysis By Product Type (Menstrual Care Products and Cleaning & Deodorizing Products), By Distribution Channel (Hypermarkets/Supermarkets, Convenience Stores, Drug Stores, and Others), and Regional Forecast, 2024-2032," accessed April 11, 2024. https://www.fortunebusinessinsights.com/feminine-hygiene-products-market-103530.

20 Barreto, Brittany, Megan Fuller, Ariella Tal, Saumya Bhatia, Jennifer Ma, Disha Trivedi, Cristy Gross, Anna-Maria Strasser, and Alexandria Farmer. 2024. *2023 FemTech Landscape Report*, FemHealth Insights. https://www.femhealthinsights.com/reports/p/2023-femtech-landscape-report.

21 Al-Hafez, "Can genetic testing explain the cause of recurrent miscarriages?"

22 Elmore, Alex. 2023. "States That Require Free Period Products In Schools." *Aunt Flow*. Updated August 1, 2023. https://goauntflow.com/blog/states-access-to-period-products-in-schools/.

## Chapter 2

23 World Health Organization. 2023. "Endometriosis." March 24, 2023. https://www.who.int/news-room/fact-sheets/detail/endometriosis.

24 Polak, Grzegorz, Beata Banaszewska, Michał Filip, Michał Radwan, Artur Wdowiak, and Paul B. Tchounwou. 2021. "Environmental Factors and Endometriosis." *International Journal of Environmental Research and Public Health* 18, no. 21: 11025. https://doi.org/10.3390/ijerph182111025.

25 Dessouky, Riham, Sherif A. Gamil, Mohamad Gamal Nada, Rola Mousa, and Yasmine Libda. 2019. "Management of uterine adenomyosis: current trends and uterine artery embolization as a potential alternative to hysterectomy." *Insights into Imaging* 10, no. 48. https://doi.org/10.1186/s13244-019-0732-8.

26 Baker, Valerie. n.d. "Uterine Fibroids: Q&A With an Expert." Johns Hopkins Medicine, accessed April 11, 2023. https://www.hopkinsmedicine.org/health/conditions-and-diseases/uterine-fibroids-qa-with-an-expert.

27 American Cancer Society. 2024. "Key Statistics for Endometrial Cancer." January 17, 2024. https://www.cancer.org/cancer/types/endometrial-cancer/about/key-statistics.html.

28 World Cancer Research Fund International. 2022. "Endometrial cancer statistics." March 23, 2022. https://www.wcrf.org/cancer-trends/endometrial-cancer-statistics/.

29 Acién, Pedro, and Irene Velasco. 2013. "Endometriosis: A Disease That Remains Enigmatic." *ISRN Obstetrics and Gynecology*, no. 1: 242149. https://doi.org/10.1155/2013/242149.

30 Planned Parenthood South, East, and North Florida. 2021. "The History of Hysteria and How it Impacts You." July 9, 2021. https://www.plannedparenthood.org/planned-parenthood-south-east-north-florida/blog/the-history-of-hysteria-and-how-it-impacts-you.

31 Frankel, Lexi. 2022. "A 10-Year Journey to Diagnosis With Endometriosis: An Autobiographical Case Report." *Cureus* 14, no. 1: e21329. https://doi.org/10.7759/cureus.21329.

32 Chaichian, Shahla. 2019. "It Is the Time to Treat Endometriosis Based on Pathophysiology." *Journal of Reproduction & Infertility* 20, no. 1: 1-2. https://www.ncbi.nlm.nih.gov/pmc/articles/PMC6386790/.

## Chapter 3

33 Leyva-Gómez, Gerardo, María L Del Prado-Audelo, Silvestre Ortega-Peña, Néstor Mendoza-Muñoz, Zaida Urbán-Morlán, Maykel González-Torres, Manuel González-Del Carmen, Gabriela Figueroa-González, Octavio D Reyes-Hernández, and Hernán Cortés. 2019. "Modifications in Vaginal Microbiota and Their Influence on Drug Release: Challenges and Opportunities." *Pharmaceutics* 11, no. 5: 217. https://doi.org/10.3390/pharmaceutics11050217.

34 Sim, Michelle, Susan Logan, and Lay Hoon Goh. 2020. "Vaginal discharge: evaluation and management in primary care." *Singapore Medical Journal* 61, no. 6: 297-301. https://doi.org/10.11622/smedj.2020088.

35 LeWine, Howard. 2023. "Vaginal yeast infection." Harvard Medical School, Harvard Health Publishing. September 21, 2023. https://www.health.harvard.edu/a_to_z/vaginal-yeast-infection-a-to-z.

36 Muzny, Christina A., and Jane R. Schwebke. 2020. "Asymptomatic Bacterial Vaginosis: To Treat or Not to Treat?" Current Infectious Disease Reports 22, no. 12: 32. https://doi.org/10.1007/s11908-020-00740-z.

37 World Health Organization. 2023. "Sexually transmitted infections (STIs)." May 21, 2024. https://www.who.int/news-room/fact-sheets/detail/sexually-transmitted-infections-(stis).

38 American Sexual Health Association. n.d. "Understanding Women's Experiences with Bacterial Vaginosis," accessed April 11, 2023. https://www.ashasexualhealth.org/understanding-womens-experiences-with-bacterial-vaginosis.

39 Medina, Martha, and Edgardo Castillo-Pino. 2019. "An introduction to the epidemiology and burden of urinary tract infections." *Therapeutic Advances in Urology* 11. https://doi.org/10.1177/1756287219832172.

40 Wei Tan, Chee, and Maciej Piotr Chlebicki. 2016. "Urinary tract infections in adults." *Singapore Medical Journal* 57, no. 9: 485-490. https://doi.org/10.11622/smedj.2016153.

41 Arnold, James, Laura Hehn, and David Klein. 2016. "Common Questions About Recurrent Urinary Tract Infections in Women." *American Family Physician* 93, no. 7: 560-569. https://www.aafp.org/pubs/afp/issues/2016/0401/p560.html

42 Zota, Ami R., and Bhavna Shamasunder. 2017. "The environmental injustice of beauty: framing chemical exposures from beauty products as a health disparities concern." *American Journal of Obstetrics and Gynecology* 217, no. 4: 418.e1–418.e6. https://doi.org/10.1016/j.ajog.2017.07.020.

43 Singh, Jessica, Sunni L. Mumford, Anna Z. Pollack, Enrique F. Schisterman, Marc G. Weisskopf, Ana Navas-Acien, and Marianthi-Anna Kioumourtzoglou. 2019. "Tampon use, environmental chemicals and oxidative stress in the BioCycle study." *Environmental Health* 18, no. 11. https://doi.org/10.1186/s12940-019-0452-z.

44 Zota, Ami, Elissia T. Franklin, Emily B. Weaver, Bhavna Shamasunder, Astrid Williams, Eva L. Siegel, and Robin E. Dodson. 2023. "Examining differences in menstrual and intimate care product use by race/ethnicity and education among menstruating individuals." *Frontiers in Reproductive Health* 5, 1286920. https://doi.org/10.3389/frph.2023.1286920.

## Chapter 4

45 Andrejek, Nicole, Tina Fetner, and Melanie Heath. 2022. "Climax as Work: Heteronormativity, Gender Labor, and the Gender Gap in Orgasms." *Gender & Society* 36, no. 2: 189-213. https://doi.org/10.1177/08912432211073062.

46 Rosen, Raymond C. 2000. "Prevalence and risk factors of sexual dysfunction in men and women." *Current Psychiatry Reports* 2, no. 3: 189-195. https://doi.org/10.1007/s11920-996-0006-2.

## Chapter 5

47 Children's Hospital of Philadelphia. 2019. "Managing Menstruation with Hormonal Contraceptives." November 19, 2019. https://www.chop.edu/news/health-tip/managing-menstruation-hormonal-contraceptives.

48 Planned Parenthood. n.d. "What are the side effects of IUDs?" Accessed April 12, 2024. https://www.plannedparenthood.org/learn/birth-control/iud/iud-side-effects.

49 Committee on Health Care for Underserved Women. 2015. "Access to Contraception." The American College of Obstetrics and Gynecologists. January 2015. https://www.acog.org/clinical/clinical-guidance/committee-opinion/articles/2015/01/access-to-contraception.

## Chapter 6

50 World Health Organization. 2023. "Infertility." April 3, 2023. https://www.who.int/news-room/fact-sheets/detail/infertility.

51 World Health Organization. 2023. "1 in 6 people globally affected by infertility: WHO." April 4, 2023.) https://www.who.int/news/item/04-04-2023-1-in-6-people-globally-affected-by-infertility.

52 Tang, Jing, Yun Xu, Zhaorui Wang, Xiaohui Ji, Qi Qiu, Zhuoyao Mai, Jia Huang, Nengyong Ouyang, and Hui Chen. 2023. "Association between metabolic healthy obesity and female infertility: the national health and nutrition examination survey, 2013–2020." *BMC Public Health* 23, no. 1: 1524. https://doi.org/10.1186/s12889-023-16397-x.

53 Sharma, Rakesh, Kelly R. Biedenharn, Jennifer M. Fedor, and Ashok Agarwal. 2013. "Lifestyle factors and reproductive health: taking control of your fertility." *Reproductive Biology and Endocrinology* 11, no. 1: 66. https://doi.org/10.1186/1477-7827-11-66.

54 Joseph, Dana N. and Shannon Whirledge. 2017. "Stress and the HPA Axis: Balancing Homeostasis and Fertility." *International Journal of Molecular Sciences* 18, no. 10: 2224. https://doi.org/10.3390/ijms18102224.

55 Silvestris, Erica, Giovanni de Pergola, Raffaele Rosania, and Giuseppe Loverro. 2018. "Obesity as disruptor of the female fertility." *Reproductive Biology and Endocrinology* 16, no. 1: 22. https://doi.org/10.1186/s12958-018-0336-z.

56 Chiang, Catheryne, Sharada Mahalingam, and Jodi A. Flaws. 2017. "Environmental Contaminants Affecting Fertility and Somatic Health." *Seminars in Reproductive Medicine* 35, no. 3: 241-249. https://doi.org/10.1055/s-0037-1603569.

57 Delbaere, Ilse, Sarah Verbiest, and Tanja Tydén. 2020. "Knowledge about the impact of age on fertility: a brief review." *Upsala Journal of Medical Sciences* 125, no. 2: 167-174. https://doi.org/10.1080/03009734.2019.1707913.

58 The Practice Committee of the American Society for Reproductive Medicine. 2014. "Female Age-Related Fertility Decline." The American College of Obstetrics and Gynecologists, last modified 2022. https://www.acog.org/clinical/clinical-guidance/committee-opinion/articles/2014/03/female-age-related-fertility-decline.

59 World Health Organization. 2023. "Polycystic ovary syndrome." June 28, 2023. https://www.who.int/news-room/fact-sheets/detail/polycystic-ovary-syndrome.

60 Johns Hopkins Medicine. n.d. "Endometriosis," accessed April 12, 2024. https://www.hopkinsmedicine.org/health/conditions-and-diseases/endometriosis.

61 Babakhanzadeh, Emad, Majid Nazari, Sina Ghasemifar, and Ali Khodadadian. 2020. "Some of the Factors Involved in Male Infertility: A Prospective Review." *International Journal of General Medicine* 13, 29-41. https://doi.org/10.2147/IJGM.S241099.

62 WHO, "1 in 6 people globally affected by infertility: WHO."

## Chapter 7

63 Soma-Pillay, Priya, Catherine Nelson-Piercy, Heli Tolppanen, and Alexandre Mebazaa. 2016. "Physiological changes in pregnancy." *Cardiovascular Journal of Africa* 27, no. 2: 89-94. https://doi.org/10.5830/CVJA-2016-021.

64 Centers for Disease Control and Prevention. 2024. "Working Together to Reduce Black Maternal Mortality." April 8, 2024. https://www.cdc.gov/healthequity/features/maternal-mortality/index.html.

65 Centers for Disease Control and Prevention. 2022. "Disparities and Resilience Among American Indian and Alaska Native People who are Pregnant or Postpartum." November 16, 2022. https://www.cdc.gov/hearher/aian/disparities.html.

66 Fischer, Barbara, and Philipp Mitteroecker. 2015. "Covariation between human pelvis shape, stature, and head size alleviates the obstetric dilemma." *Proceedings of the National Academy of Sciences* 112, no. 18: 5655–5660. https://doi.org/10.1073/pnas.1420325112.

67 Birth Injury Help Center. n.d. "The History of Childbirth," accessed April 13, 2024. https://www.birthinjuryhelpcenter.org/childbirth-history.html.

68 National Health Service. n.d. "Miscarriage," accessed April 13, 2024. https://www.nhs.uk/conditions/miscarriage/.

69 Vlachadis, Nikolaos, Theti Papadopoulou, Dionysios Vrachnis, Emmanuel Manolakos, Nikolaos Loukas, Panagiotis Christopoulos, Kalliopi Pappa, and Nikolaos Vrachnis. 2023. "Incidence and Types of Chromosomal Abnormalities in First Trimester Spontaneous Miscarriages: a Greek Single-Center Prospective Study." *Mœdica* 18, no. 1: 35-41. https://doi.org/10.26574/maedica.2023.18.1.35.

70 Ibid.

71 Wisner, Katherine, Dorothy Sit, Mary McShea, David Rizzo, Rebecca Zoretich, Carolyn Hughes, Heather Eng, James Luther, Stephen Wisniewski, Michelle Costantino, Andrea Confer, Eydie Moses-Kolko, Christopher Famy, and Barbara Hanusa. 2013. "Onset Timing, Thoughts of Self-harm, and Diagnoses in Postpartum Women With Screen-Positive Depression Findings." *JAMA Psychiatry* 70, no. 5: 490-498. https://doi.org/10.1001/jamapsychiatry.2013.87.

72 World Health Organization. 2021. "Caesarean section rates continue to rise, amid growing inequalities in access." June 16, 2021. https://www.who.int/news/item/16-06-2021-caesarean-section-rates-continue-to-rise-amid-growing-inequalities-in-access.

73 Ibid.

74 Ibid.

75 World Health Organization. 2023. "Maternal mortality." February 22, 2023. https://www.who.int/news-room/fact-sheets/detail/maternal-mortality.

76 Katella, Kathy. 2023. "Maternal Mortality Is on the Rise: 8 Things To Know." Yale Medicine. May 22, 2023. https://www.yalemedicine.org/news/maternal-mortality-on-the-rise.

77 Hoyert, Donna. 2023. "Maternal Mortality Rates in the United States, 2021." Centers for Disease Control and Prevention. March 16, 2023. https://www.cdc.gov/nchs/data/hestat/maternal-mortality/2021/maternal-mortality-rates-2021.htm.

78 World Health Organization. n.d. "Abortion," accessed April 13, 2024. https://www.who.int/health-topics/abortion.

79 Planned Parenthood. n.d. "How safe is the abortion pill?" Accessed May 22, 2024. https://www.plannedparenthood.org/learn/abortion/the-abortion-pill/how-safe-is-the-abortion-pill.

80 World Health Organization. 2021. "Abortion." Newsroom, updated May 17, 2024. https://www.who.int/news-room/fact-sheets/detail/abortion.

## Chapter 8

81 Centers for Disease Control and Prevention. 2023. "About Breastfeeding." December 18, 2023. https://www.cdc.gov/breastfeeding/php/about/?CDC_AAref_Val=https://www.cdc.gov/breastfeeding/about-breastfeeding/why-it-matters.html.

82 Ibid.

83 Tauber, Kate A. 2021. "Human Milk and Lactation." *Medscape*. June 29, 2021. https://emedicine.medscape.com/article/1835675-overview?form=fpf#showall.

84 Ibid.

85 Centers for Disease Control and Prevention. n.d. "Rates of Any and Exclusive Breastfeeding by Socio-demographics among Children Born in 2020," accessed April 22, 2024. https://www.cdc.gov/breastfeeding/data/nis_data/rates-any-exclusive-bf-socio-dem-2020.htm.

86 Quintero, Stephanie M., Paula D. Strassle, Amalia Londoño Tobón, Stephanie Ponce, Alia Alhomsi, Ana I. Maldonado, Jamie S. Ko, Miciah J Wilkerson, and Anna María Nápoles. 2023. "Race/ethnicity-specific associations between breastfeeding information source and breastfeeding rates among U.S. women." *BMC Public Health* 23, no. 1: 520. https://doi.org/10.1186/s12889-023-15447-8.

87 Asiodu, Ifeyinwa V., Kimarie Bugg, and Aunchalee E. L. Palmquist. 2021. "Achieving Breastfeeding Equity and Justice in Black Communities: Past, Present, and Future." *Breastfeeding Medicine* 16, no. 6: 447–451. https://doi.org/10.1089/bfm.2020.0314.

88 Brown, Amy. 2020. "9 Sociological and Cultural Influences upon Breastfeeding." *In Breastfeeding and Breast Milk—from Biochemistry to Impact.* The Global Health Network. May 1, 2020. https://doi.org/10.21428/3d48c34a.2a0f254a.

## Chapter 9

89 UCLA Health. n.d. "Pelvic floor disorders." Urogynecology & Pelvic Health, accessed April 13, 2024. https://www.uclahealth.org/medical-services/womens-pelvic-health/patient-education/pelvic-floor-disorders.

90 Adriana Peinado-Molina, Rocío, Antonio Hernández-Martínez, Sergio Martínez-Vázquez, Julián Rodríguez-Almagro, and Juan Miguel Martínez-Galiano. 2023. "Pelvic floor dysfunction: prevalence and associated factors." *BMC Public Health* 23, no. 1: 2005. https://doi.org/10.1186/s12889-023-16901-3.

91 European Association of Urology. 2023. "The annual economic burden of urinary incontinence could reach €87 billion in 2030 if no action is taken." November 8, 2023. https://uroweb.org/press-releases/the-annual-economic-burden-of-urinary-incontinence-could-reach-87-billion-in-2030-if-no-action-is-taken.

92 St. Martin, Brad, Melissa A. Markowitz, Evan R. Myers, Lisbet S. Lundsberg, and Nancy Ringel. 2024. "Estimated National Cost of Pelvic Organ Prolapse Surgery in the United States." *Obstetrics & Gynecology* 143, no. 3: 419-427. https://doi.org/10.1097/AOG.0000000000005485.

## Chapter 10

93 National Institute on Aging. 2021. "What is Menopause?" National Institutes of Health. September 30, 2021. https://www.nia.nih.gov/health/menopause/what-menopause.

94 Mayo Clinic. 2023. "Menopause." May 25, 2023. https://www.mayoclinic.org/diseases-conditions/menopause/symptoms-causes/syc-20353397.

95 Christianson, Mindy S., Jennifer A. Ducie, Kristiina Altman, Ayatallah M. Khafagy, and Wen Shen. 2013. "Menopause education: needs assessment of American obstetrics and gynecology residents." *Menopause* 20, no. 11: 1120-1125. https://doi.org/10.1097/GME.0b013e31828ced7f.

96 Kopenhager, T., and F. Guidozzi. 2015. "Working women and the menopause." Climacteric: The Journal of the International Menopause Society 18, no. 3: 372–375. https://doi.org/10.3109/13697137.2015.1020483.

97 Biote. *Biote Women in the Workplace Survey*. 2022. https://biote.com/learning-center/biote-women-in-the-workplace-survey.

98 Furst, Jay. 2023. "Mayo Clinic study puts price tag on cost of menopause symptoms for women in the workplace." *Mayo Clinic.* April 26, 2023. https://newsnetwork.mayoclinic.org/discussion/mayo-clinic-study-puts-price-tag-on-cost-of-menopause-symptoms-for-women-in-the-workplace/.

99 *Biote Women in the Workplace Survey.*

100 Ibid.

101 Ibid.

102 Barreto, Brittany, Megan Fuller, Ariella Tal, Saumya Bhatia, Jennifer Ma, Disha Trivedi, Cristy Gross, Anna-Maria Strasser, and Alexandria Farmer. 2024. *2023*

*FemTech Landscape Report*, FemHealth Insights. https://www.femhealthinsights.com/reports/p/2023-femtech-landscape-report.

103 Bhatia, Saumya. 2024. *Menopause Minireport*, FemHealth Insights. https://www.femhealthinsights.com/reports/p/menopause.

## Chapter 11

104 American Cancer Society. n.d. "All About Cancer," accessed April 18, 2024. https://www.cancer.org/cancer.html.

105 American Cancer Society. 2024. "Key Statistics for Breast Cancer." January 17, 2024. https://www.cancer.org/cancer/types/breast-cancer/about/how-common-is-breast-cancer.html.

106 Breastcancer.org. 2024. "Breast Cancer Facts and Statistics," updated May 22, 2024. https://www.breastcancer.org/facts-statistics

107 Ibid.

108 Ibid.

109 Penn Medicine. 2021. "What Women Need to Know About Lung Cancer." October 7, 2021. https://www.pennmedicine.org/cancer/about/focus-on-cancer/2021/october/lung-cancer-what-women-should-know.

110 Gazdar, Adi F., Sophie Sun, and Joan H. Schiller. 2007. "Lung cancer in never smokers—a different disease." Nature Reviews Cancer 7, no. 10: 778–790. https://doi.org/10.1038/nrc2190.

111 Women's Health Access Matters. n.d. "The Case to Fund Women's Health Research," accessed April 18, 2024. https://thewhamreport.org/report/.

112 Spencer, Ryan J., Laurel W. Rice, Clara Ye, Kaitlin Woo, and Shitanshu Uppal. 2019. "Disparities in the Allocation of Research Funding to Gynecologic Cancers by Funding to Lethality Scores." *Gynecologic Oncology* 152, no. 1: 106–111. https://doi.org/10.1016/j.ygyno.2018.10.021.

113 Winstead, Edward. 2022. "Severe Side Effects of Cancer Treatment Are More Common in Women than Men." National Cancer Institute. March 15, 2022. https://www.cancer.gov/news-events/cancer-currents-blog/2022/cancer-treatment-women-severe-side-effects.

114 Unger, Joseph M., Riha Vaidya, Kathy S. Albain, Michael LeBlanc, Lori M. Minasian, Carolyn C. Gotay, N. Lynn Henry, Michael J. Fisch, Shing M. Lee, Charles D. Blanke, and Dawn L. Hershman. 2022. "Sex Differences in Risk of Severe Adverse Events in Patients Receiving Immunotherapy, Targeted Therapy, or Chemotherapy in Cancer Clinical Trials." *Journal of Clinical Oncology* 40, no. 13: 1474-1486. https://doi.org/10.1200/JCO.21.02377.

115 McKinsey & Company. 2022. "Unlocking opportunities in women's healthcare." February 14, 2022. https://www.mckinsey.com/industries/healthcare/our-insights/unlocking-opportunities-in-womens-healthcare.

116 Ibid.

117 Spencer, "Disparities in the Allocation of Research Funding to Gynecologic Cancers by Funding to Lethality Scores."

118 Arasu, Vignesh A., Laurel A. Habel, Ninah S. Achacoso, Diana S. M. Buist, Jason B. Cord, Laura J. Esserman, Nola M. Hylton, M. Maria Glymour, John Kornak, Lawrence H. Kushi, Donald A. Lewis, Vincent X. Liu, Caitlin M. Lydon, Diana L. Miglioretti, Daniel A. Navarro, Albert Pu, Li Shen, Weiva Sieh, Hyo-Chun Yoon, and Catherine Lee. 2023. "Comparison of Mammography AI Algorithms with a Clinical Risk Model for 5-year Breast Cancer Risk Prediction: An Observational Study." *Radiology* 307, no. 5. https://doi.org/10.1148/radiol.222733.

119 Arasu, "Comparison of Mammography AI Algorithms with a Clinical Risk Model for 5-year Breast Cancer Risk Prediction: An Observational Study."

120 Centers for Disease Control and Prevention. 2023. "Mammography." June 26, 2023. https://www.cdc.gov/nchs/hus/topics/mammography.htm.

121 Susan G. Komen. 2024. "How Do Breast Cancer Screening Rates Compare Among Different Groups in the U.S.?" January 23, 2024. https://www.komen.org/breast-cancer/screening/screening-disparities/

122 MSD Manual Professional Edition. 2023. "Benign Ovarian Masses." Retrieved from MSD Manuals

## Chapter 12

123 Komagamine, Tomoko, Norito Kokubun, and Koichi Hirata. 2020. "Battey's operation as a treatment for hysteria: a review of a series of cases in the nineteenth century." History of psychiatry 31, no. 1: 55–66. https://doi.org/10.1177/0957154X19877145.

124 Gogos, Andrea, Luke J. Ney, Natasha Seymour, Tamsyn E. Van Rheenen, and Kim L. Felmingham. 2019. "Sex differences in schizophrenia, bipolar disorder, and post-traumatic stress disorder: are gonadal hormones the link?" *British Journal of Pharmacology* 176, no. 21: 4119–4135. https://doi.org/10.1111/bph.14584.

125 *Youth Risk Behavior Survey: Data Summary & Trends Report: 2011-2021*, Centers for Disease Control and Prevention, 2023. https://www.cdc.gov/healthyyouth/data/yrbs/pdf/yrbs_data-summary-trends_report2023_508.pdf.

126 Substance Abuse and Mental Health Services Administration. 2021. *Key Substance Use and Mental Health Indicators in the United States: Results from the 2020 National Survey on Drug Use and Health*, US Department of Health and Human Services. https://store.samhsa.gov/.

127 U.S. Department of Veterans Affairs. 2022. "Military Sexual Trauma," accessed September 22, 2022. https://www.ptsd.va.gov/understand/types/sexual_trauma_military.asp.

## Chapter 13

128 Raghupathi, Wullianallur, and Viju Raghupathi. 2018. "An Empirical Study of Chronic Diseases in the United States: A Visual Analytics Approach to Public Health." *International Journal of Environmental Research and Public Health* 15, no. 3: 431. https://doi.org/10.3390/ijerph15030431.

129 Temkin, Sarah M., Elizabeth Barr, Holly Moore, Juliane P. Caviston, Judith G. Regensteiner, and Janine A. Clayton. 2023. "Chronic conditions in women: the development of a National Institutes of Health framework." *BMC Women's Health* 23, no. 1: 162. https://doi.org/10.1186/s12905-023-02319-x.

130 Moretti, Chiara, Enrico De Luca, Clelia D'Apice, Giovanna Artioli, Leopoldo Sarli, and Antonio Bonacaro. 2023. "Gender and sex bias in prevention and clinical treatment of women's chronic pain: hypotheses of a curriculum development." *Frontiers in Medicine* 10, 1189126. https://doi.org/10.3389/fmed.2023.1189126.

131 Boersma, Peter, Lindsey I. Black, and Brian W. Ward. 2020. "Prevalence of Multiple Chronic Conditions Among US Adults, 2018." *Preventing Chronic Disease 17*: E106. https://doi.org/10.5888/pcd17.200130.

132 Temkin, "Chronic conditions in women: the development of a National Institutes of Health framework."

133 Jo, Eun-Jung, Young Uk Lee, Ahreum Kim, Hye-Kyung Park, and Changhoon Kim. 2023. "The prevalence of multiple chronic conditions and medical burden in asthma patients." *PloS one* 18, no. 5: e0286004. https://doi.org/10.1371/journal.pone.0286004.

134 Centers for Medicare & Medicaid Services (CMS). "Chronic Conditions among Medicare Beneficiaries: A Methodological Overview.". 2020. https://www.cms.gov/Research-Statistics-Data-and-Systems/Statistics-Trends-and-Reports/Chronic-Conditions/Downloads/Methods_Overview.pdf.

135 Temkin, "Chronic conditions in women: the development of a National Institutes of Health framework."

136 Kronzer, Vanessa L., Stanley Louis Bridges, and John M. Davis. 2021. "Why women have more autoimmune diseases than men: an evolutionary perspective." *Evolutionary Applications* 14, no. 3: 629–633. https://doi.org/10.1111/eva.13167.

137 Merone, Lea, Komla Tsey, Darren Russell, Andrew Daltry, and Cate Nagle. 2022. "Self-Reported Time to Diagnosis and Proportions of Rediagnosis in Female Patients with Chronic Conditions in Australia: A Cross-sectional Survey." *Women's Health Reports* 3, no. 1: 749–758. https://doi.org/10.1089/whr.2022.0040.

138 Westergaard, David, Pope Moseley, Freja Karuna Hemmingsen Sørup, Pierre Baldi, and Søren Brunak. 2019. "Population-Wide Analysis of Differences in Disease Progression Patterns in Men and Women." *Nature Communications* 10, no. 1: 666. https://doi.org/10.1038/s41467-019-08475-9.

139 Novo Nordisk Foundation Center for Protein Research. 2019. *Study: Across Diseases, Women Are Diagnosed Later Than Men.* March 10, 2019. https://www.cpr.ku.dk/cpr-news/2019/study-across-diseases-women-are-diagnosed-later-than-men/.

140 Miller, Jennifer. 2022. "Women + Chronic Illness: Still Waiting to Be Heard." Health Central. March 24, 2022. https://www.healthcentral.com/article/women-and-chronic-disease.

141 Ibid.

142 Federation of State Medical Boards. 2019. "National Survey Indicates Majority of Physician Misconduct Goes Unreported." May 30, 2019. https://www.fsmb.org/advocacy/news-releases/national-survey-indicates-majority-of-physician-misconduct-goes-unreported.

143 Miller, "Women + Chronic Illness: Still Waiting to Be Heard."

144 Miller, "Women + Chronic Illness: Still Waiting to Be Heard."

145 Miller, "Women + Chronic Illness: Still Waiting to Be Heard."

146 Miller, "Women + Chronic Illness: Still Waiting to Be Heard."

147 Johnson, Pamela Jo, Judy Jou, and Dawn M. Upchurch. 2020. "Psychological Distress and Access to Care Among Midlife Women." *Journal of Aging and Health* 32, no. 5–6: 317–327. https://doi.org/10.1177/0898264318822367.

148 Harvard Health Blog. 2017. "Women and pain: Disparities in experience and treatment." October 9, 2017. https://www.health.harvard.edu/blog/women-and-pain-disparities-in-experience-and-treatment-2017100912562#.

149 Hoffmann, Diane E., and Anita J. Tarzian. 2021. "The Girl Who Cried Pain: A Bias Against Women in the Treatment of Pain." *The Journal of Law, Medicine & Ethics* 29, no. 1: 13–27. https://doi.org/10.1111/j.1748-720X.2001.tb00037.x.

150 Dahlhamer, James, Jacqueline Lucas, Carla Zelaya, Richard Nahin, Sean Mackey, Lynn DeBar, Robert Kerns, Michael Von Korff, Linda Porter, and Charles Helmick. 2018. "Prevalence of Chronic Pain and High-Impact Chronic Pain Among Adults—United States, 2016." *Morbidity and Mortality Weekly Report* 67, no. 36: 1001–1006. https://doi.org/10.15585/mmwr.mm6736a2.

151 Ibid.

152 Latifi, Fortesa. "The Pain Gap: Why Women's Pain Is Undertreated." *HealthyWomen*, July 26, 2021. https://www.healthywomen.org/condition/pain-gap-womens-pain-undertreated.

153 Ibid.

154 Hoffman, Kelly M., Sophie Trawalter, Jordan R. Axt, and M. Norman Oliver. 2016. "Racial bias in pain assessment and treatment recommendations, and false beliefs about biological differences between blacks and whites." *Proceedings of the National Academy of Sciences* 113, no. 16: 4296–4301. https://doi.org/10.1073/pnas.1516047113.

155 King Edward VII's Hospital. n.d. "6 million await diagnosis for women's health conditions," accessed April 20, 2024. https://www.kingedwardvii.co.uk/about-king-edward-vii/news/6-million-await-diagnosis-for-womens-health-conditions.

## Chapter 14

156 Jacobs, Emily G., 2023. "Only 0.5% of neuroscience studies look at women's health. Here's how to change that." *Nature* 623, no. 7988: 667-667. https://doi.org/10.1038/d41586-023-03614-1.

157 Weill Cornell Medicine Neurology. n.d. "Women's Brain Initiative," accessed May 1, 2024. https://neurology.weill.cornell.edu/research/womens-brain-initiative.

158 Ibid.

159 Lohner, Valerie, Gökhan Pehlivan, Gerard Sanroma, Anne Miloschewski, Markus D. Schirmer, Tony Stöcker, Martin Reuter, and Monique M.B. Breteler. 2022. "Relation Between Sex, Menopause, and White Matter Hyperintensities." *Neurology Journals* 99, no. 9: e935-e943. https://doi.org/10.1212/WNL.0000000000200782.

160 Bone Health & Osteoporosis Foundation. n.d. "What Women Need to Know," accessed May 1, 2024. https://www.bonehealthandosteoporosis.org/preventing-fractures/general-facts/what-women-need-to-know/.

161 Bone Health & Osteoporosis Foundation. n.d. "Osteoporosis Fast Facts," accessed May 1, 2024. https://www.bonehealthandosteoporosis.org/wp-content/uploads/Osteoporosis-Fast-Facts-2.pdf.

162 Swift, Diana. n.d. "The High Cost of Osteoporosis." Medpage Today. Accessed May 1, 2024. https://www.medpagetoday.com/medical-journeys/osteoporosis/108129.

163 Bone Health & Osteoporosis Foundation, "Osteoporosis Fact Sheet."

164 Ibid.

[165] Schattner, Amy. 2018. "The burden of hip fractures—why aren't we better at prevention?" *QJM: An International Journal of Medicine* 111, no. 11: 765-767. https://doi.org/10.1093/qjmed/hcx216.

166 Centers for Disease Control and Prevention. 2024. "About Women and Heart Disease." May 15, 2024. https://www.cdc.gov/heart-disease/about/women-and-heart-disease.html?CDC_AAref_Val=https://www.cdc.gov/heartdisease/women.htm.

167 Ibid.

168 Ibid.

169 Mu, Fan, Janet Rich-Edwards, Eric Rimm, Donna Spiegelman, and Stacey Missmer. 2016."Endometriosis and Risk of Coronary Heart Disease." *Circulation: Cardiovascular Quality and Outcomes* 9, no. 3: 257–264. https://doi.org/10.1161/circoutcomes.115.002224.

170 Sauer, Emma. 2022. "The Gender Gap in Caregiving and Why Women Carry It." University of Missouri-Kansas City Women's Center. March 9, 2022. https://info.umkc.edu/womenc/2022/03/09/the-gender-gap-in-caregiving-and-why-women-carry-it/.

171 National Center on Caregiving at Family Caregiver Alliance. n.d. "Women and Caregiving: Facts and Figures," accessed May 1, 2024. https://www.caregiver.org/resource/women-and-caregiving-facts-and-figures/.

172 Ibid.

173 Alon, Titan, Matthias Doepke, Jane Olmstead-Rumsey, and Michèle Tertilt. 2020. "The Impact of COVID-19 on Gender Equality." *IDEAS Working Paper Series from RePEc*. https://www.nber.org/system/files/working_papers/w26947/w26947.pdf.

174 Cannuscio, Carolyn C, Camara Jones, Ichiro Kawachi, Graham A Colditz, Lisa Berkman, and Eric Rimm. 2002. "Reverberations of Family Illness: A Longitudinal Assessment of Informal Caregiving and Mental Health Status in the Nurses' Health Study." *American Journal of Public Health* 92, no. 8: 1305–1311. https://doi.org/10.2105/ajph.92.8.1305.

175 National Center on Caregiving at Family Caregiver Alliance. "Women and Caregiving: Facts and Figures

176 Cannuscio, "Reverberations of Family Illness: A Longitudinal Assessment of Informal Caregiving and Mental Health Status in the Nurses' Health Study."

## Chapter 15

177 Huh, Woonghee Tim, Jaywon Lee, Heesang Park, and Kun Soo Park. 2019. "The potty parity problem: Towards gender equality at restrooms in business facilities." *Socio-Economic Planning Sciences* 68, 100666. https://doi.org/10.1016/j.seps.2018.11.003.

178 Basager, Ahmed, Quintin Williams, Rosie Hanneke, Aishwarya Sanaka, and Heather M. Weinreich. 2024. "Musculoskeletal disorders and discomfort for female surgeons or surgeons with small hand size when using hand-held surgical instruments: a systematic review." *Systematic Reviews* 13, no. 1: 57. https://doi.org/10.1186/s13643-024-02462-y.

## Chapter 16

179 Bloom, Floyde E., and Mark A. Randolph, eds. 1990. *Funding Health Sciences Research: A Strategy to Restore Balance*. National Academies Press. https://www.ncbi.nlm.nih.gov/books/NBK235736/.

180 National Institutes of Health. 2023. "Direct Economic Contributions." *Serving Society*. December 8, 2023. https://www.nih.gov/about-nih/what-we-do/impact-nih-research/serving-society/direct-economic-contributions.

181 Mikulic, Matej. 2023. "Total women's health funding by National Institutes for Health 2013-2024." Statista. June 1, 2023. https://www.statista.com/statistics/713378/total-women-s-health-funding-by-the-national-institutes-for-health/.

182 National Institutes of Health. 2021. "NIH Awards by Location & Organization." *Research Portfolio and Online Reporting Tools (RePORT)*. January 8, 2021. https://report.nih.gov/award/index.cfm?ot=&fy=2020&state=&ic=&fm=&orgid=&distr=&rfa=&om=n&pid=.

183 Ellingrud, Kweilin, Lucy Pérez, Anouk Petersen, and Valentina Sartori. 2024. *Closing the Women's Health Gap: A $1 Trillion Opportunity to Improve Lives and Economies*, World Economic Forum. https://www.weforum.org/publications/closing-the-women-s-health-gap-a-1-trillion-opportunity-to-improve-lives-and-economies/.

184 Desai, Shailesh, Atul Munshi, and Devangi Munshi. 2021. "Gender Bias in Cardiovascular Disease Prevention, Detection, and Management, with Specific Reference to Coronary Artery Disease." *Journal of Mid-Life Health* 12, no. 1: 8–15. https://doi.org/10.4103/jmh.jmh_31_21.

185 Women's Health Access Matters. n.d. "The Case to Fund Women's Health Research," accessed May 9, 2024. https://thewhamreport.org/report/.

186 Harvard Kennedy School. n.d. "Advancing Gender Equality in Venture Capital," accessed May 9, 2024. https://www.hks.harvard.edu/centers/wappp/research/past/venture-capital-entrepreneurship.

187 Ellingrud, *Closing the Women's Health Gap: A $1 Trillion Opportunity to Improve Lives and Economies.*

188 Ibid.

189 Barreto, Brittany, Megan Fuller, Ariella Tal, Saumya Bhatia, Jennifer Ma, Disha Trivedi, Cristy Gross, Anna-Maria Strasser, and Alexandria Farmer. 2024. *2023 FemTech Landscape Report*, FemHealth Insights. https://www.femhealthinsights.com/reports/p/2023-femtech-landscape-report.

190 Stefanuto, Lucia. 2023. "Only 15% of Tech Startup Founders Are Female." *Startup Genome*. March 27, 2023. https://startupgenome.com/articles/only-15-percent-of-tech-startup-founders-are-female.

191 Abouzahr, Katie Matt Krentz, John Harthorne, and Frances Brooks Taplett. 2018. "Why Women-Owned Startups Are a Better Bet." *Boston Consulting Group*. June 6, 2018. https://www.bcg.com/publications/2018/why-women-owned-startups-are-better-bet.

192 Harvard Kennedy School, "Advancing Gender Equity in Venture Capital."

193 Krentz, "Why Women-Owned Startups Are a Better Bet."

## Conclusion

194 Boughton, Rebecca S., Caroline Brophy, Gillian Corbett, Sophie Murphy, Jacqui Clifford, Ann Hanly, Myra Fitzpatrick, and Laoise O'Brien. 2024. "Haemorrhoids and Anal Fissures in Pregnancy: Predictive Factors and Effective Treatments." *Cureus* 16, no. 2: e53773. https://doi.org/10.7759/cureus.53773.

195 Bernstein, Matthew T., Lesley A. Graff, Lisa Avery, Carrie Palatnick, Katie Parnerowski, and Laura E. Targownik. 2014. "Gastrointestinal symptoms before and during menses in healthy women." *BMC Women's Health* 14, no. 14. https://doi.org/10.1186/1472-6874-14-14.

196 United Nations Office for Outer Space Affairs. n.d. "About Space4Women." *Space4Women*, accessed May 28, 2024. https://space4women.unoosa.org/about.

197 Fortin, Jacey, and Karen Zraick. 2019. "First All-Female Spacewalk Canceled Because NASA Doesn't Have Two Suits That Fit." *New York Times*. March 25, 2019. https://www.nytimes.com/2019/03/25/science/female-spacewalk-canceled.html.

# Acknowledgments

**I EXTEND MY DEEPEST GRATITUDE** to GracePoint Publishing. From the very beginning, you believed in my mission, even before a single word was written. Your patience, kindness, and unwavering support have been instrumental in elevating my book to a position of quality I never imagined possible. A special thank you to the director of publishing, Tascha Yoder, for your invaluable meetings and coaching. Your guidance has been a cornerstone of this journey.

I am profoundly grateful to my femhealth fellows, Amy Keenan, Ariella Tal, and Apoorva Sudini. Your contributions were critical to the inception, completion, and refinement of this book. Your efforts and dedication have made this project a reality.

To my ever-supportive family, Kelly Barreto, Sabrina Barreto, and Alix Boulard, I am deeply thankful for your love, support, and unwavering belief in me. You have provided me with the space to vent, cry, and celebrate, and it is an amazing feeling to know that you always have my back, no matter what. Your encouragement has been my greatest source of strength, and for that, I am incredibly grateful.

Lastly, I want to express my heartfelt thanks to the FemTech innovators. Entrepreneurship and advocacy are not for the faint of heart, particularly when success also requires challenging social norms, stigma, and ancient bias. Your creativity, grit, and groundbreaking inventions are saving women's lives, and I am honored to be a platform to showcase your incredible work.

Thank you all for your unwavering support and belief in this mission.

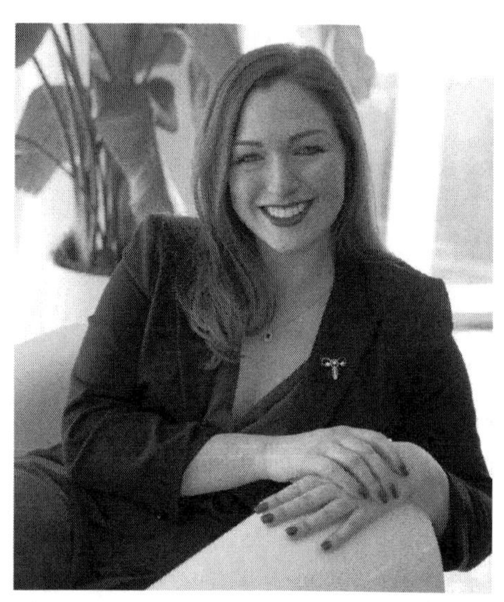

# About the Author

**DR. BRITTANY BARRETO DEDICATES HER WORK** to advancing women's health by equipping founders, investing in innovative ideas, and engaging key stakeholders to create better healthcare for women, females, and girls, an industry known as FemTech. She is the founder of FemHealth Insights, a boutique consulting firm with a market research software tool specializing in women's health innovation; host of the number one women's health innovation podcast, *FemTech Focus*; cofounder of an early-stage FemTech venture fund, Coyote Ventures; manages the largest virtual community of femtech founders, Advisory Board Member for Imperial College of London Network of Excellence in Women's Health, and identifies as an unconventional scientist, entrepreneur, and consultant who proves that anything is possible with hard work and heart.

While completing her bachelor's in biology, public health, and French at Drew University Honors College, she engaged in HHMI-funded research on potential correlations between estrogen and Alzheimer's disease, which disproportionately affects women. She then completed her doctorate at Baylor College of Medicine in molecular and human genetics, where she published her discovery of a small RNA that regulates genomic mutation rate in bacteria.

During graduate school, she founded a venture-backed startup, Pheramor, the world's first DNA-based dating app. The algorithm incorporated factors that increase sexual compatibility and fertility between matches. Another algorithm she created which predicts personality type from DNA was granted a US patent. She exited the company and shifted into investments as a senior venture associate at Texas's most active venture fund, Capital Factory.

In 2019, three years after Ida Tin coined the term FemTech, Dr. Barreto noticed how underserved the FemTech industry was and set out to bring awareness, resources, and capital to it. Today, she is considered the voice of FemTech. She has received many awards and recognitions, including a three-time recipient of Top Leaders in FemTech Award, FemForce Early Career Achievement Award, and the Young Alumni Award from Drew University. Dr. Barreto has served on women's health committees with Gates Foundation and NIH. She is invited internationally to speak on the world's largest stages about the importance of sex and gender in research and innovation. Corporations, governments, and investors revere her as the go-to women's health innovation expert.

Dr. Barreto originally hails from New Jersey and lives in Raleigh, North Carolina, with her rescue dogs, Trypsin and Quark, and guinea pig, Ginsburg. Her passions outside of FemTech include awareness for childhood trauma and complex PTSD recovery, farming, LGBTQIA+ rights, and advocating for abortion access.